# THE BEST
# IN TENT
# CAMPING

## TENNESSEE

## Other books by Johnny Molloy:

*Beach & Coastal Camping in Florida*
*The Best in Tent Camping: The Carolinas*
*The Best in Tent Camping: Colorado*
*The Best in Tent Camping: Florida*
*The Best in Tent Camping: Georgia*
*The Best in Tent Camping: Kentucky*
*The Best in Tent Camping: The Southern Appalachian & Smoky Mountains*
*The Best in Tent Camping: West Virginia*
*The Best in Tent Camping: Wisconsin*
*A Canoeing & Kayaking Guide to Florida*
*A Canoeing & Kayaking Guide to Kentucky (with Bob Sehlinger)*
*Day & Overnight Hikes: Kentucky's Sheltowee Trace*
*Day & Overnight Hikes in Shenandoah National Park*
*Day & Overnight Hikes in the Great Smoky Mountains National Park*
*From the Swamp to the Keys: A Paddle through Florida History*
*The Hiking Trails of Florida's National Forests, Parks, and Preserves*
*Land Between the Lakes Outdoor Recreation Handbook*
*Long Trails of the Southeast*
*Mount Rogers Outdoor Recreation Handbook*
*A Paddler's Guide to Everglades National Park*
*60 Hikes within 60 Miles: Nashville*
*60 Hikes within 60 Miles: San Antonio & Austin (with Tom Taylor)*
*Trial by Trail: Backpacking in the Smoky Mountains*

## Visit Johnny Molloy's Web site:
www.johnnymolloy.com

# THE BEST IN TENT CAMPING

### A GUIDE FOR CAR CAMPERS WHO HATE RVs, CONCRETE SLABS, AND LOUD PORTABLE STEREOS

## TENNESSEE

JOHNNY MOLLOY

MENASHA RIDGE PRESS
BIRMINGHAM, ALABAMA

*This book is for all my fellow Tennesseans*
*who love tent camping as much as I do.*

Copyright © 2005 by Johnny Molloy
All rights reserved
Printed in the United States of America
Published by Menasha Ridge Press
Distributed by The Globe Pequot Press
First edition, first printing

Library of Congress Cataloging in Publication
Molloy, Johnny, 1961–
    The best in tent camping, Tennessee: a guide for car campers who hate RVs, concrete slabs,
and loud portable stereos / by Johnny Molloy.—1st ed.
p.cm.
    ISBN 0-89732-608-3
    1. Camping—Tennessee—Guidebooks. 2. Camp sites, facilities, etc.—Tennessee—Directories.
    3. Tennessee—Guidebooks. I. Title.

GV191.42.T2M655 2005
796.54'09768—dc22

                                                                                    2005050521
                                                                                         CIP

Cover and text design by Palace Press International
Cover photo by Mark Carroll
Cartography by Jennie Zehmer

Menasha Ridge Press
P.O. Box 43673
Birmingham, Alabama 35243
www.menasharidge.com

# TABLE OF CONTENTS

## EAST TENNESSEE

## APPENDIXES

# MAP LEGEND

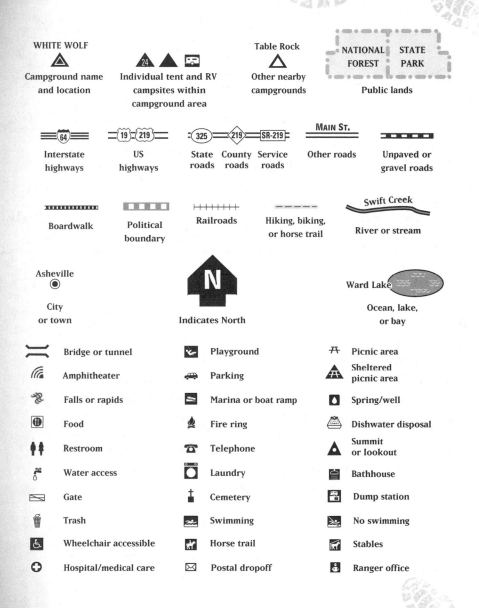

**WHITE WOLF**
Campground name
and location

Individual tent and RV
campsites within
campground area

**Table Rock**
Other nearby
campgrounds

NATIONAL FOREST | STATE PARK
Public lands

Interstate
highways

US
highways

State County Service
roads   roads   roads

**MAIN ST.**
Other roads

Unpaved or
gravel roads

Boardwalk

Political
boundary

Railroads

Hiking, biking,
or horse trail

**Swift Creek**
River or stream

**Asheville**
City
or town

**N**
Indicates North

**Ward Lake**
Ocean, lake,
or bay

Bridge or tunnel

Amphitheater

Falls or rapids

Food

Restroom

Water access

Gate

Trash

Wheelchair accessible

Hospital/medical care

Playground

Parking

Marina or boat ramp

Fire ring

Telephone

Laundry

Cemetery

Swimming

Horse trail

Postal dropoff

Picnic area

Sheltered
picnic area

Spring/well

Dishwater disposal

Summit
or lookout

Bathhouse

Dump station

No swimming

Stables

Ranger office

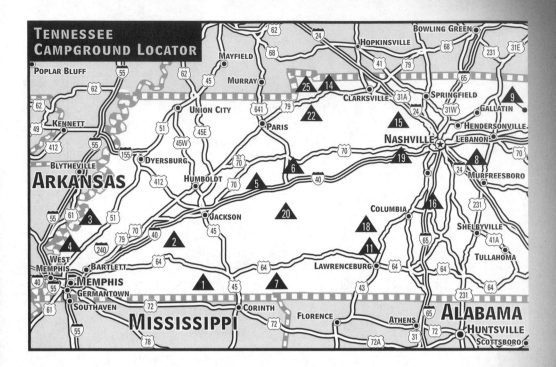

TENNESSEE CAMPGROUND LOCATOR

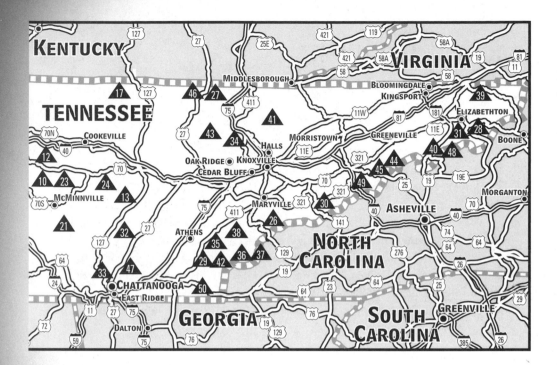

# ACKNOWLEDGMENTS

I WOULD LIKE TO THANK THE FOLLOWING people for helping me in the research and writing of this book: all the land managers of Tennessee's state parks and the folks at Land Between the Lakes, Cherokee National Forest, Great Smoky Mountains National Park, and the lakes administered by the Army Corps of Engineers.

Thanks to the innumerable friends and family members who have explored all the natural beauty of the state with me, from the west to the east. Thanks to Linda Grebe at Eureka for providing me with great tents for camping. Thanks to Silva for compasses and Camp Trails for their backpack. Thanks to Jean Cobb and the crew at Freebairn & Co.

The biggest thanks of all goes to the people of the Volunteer State, who enjoy our state from the mighty Mississippi to Mount LeConte and all points in between.

# PREFACE

**B**EING A NATIVE **T**ENNESSEAN AND **LOVER** of the outdoors, and having explored my state for 20 years, I thought I had a leg up on writing this book, knowing all I already knew about the Volunteer State. What I ended up finding out is that there is a lot more out there than I thought! Our varied topography and wealth of protected lands make for diverse outdoor venues in which to pitch a tent and then explore what makes these places so special. I currently live in Johnson City but was raised in Memphis and have lived in both Nashville and Knoxville. Between camping for fun, visiting family in Memphis, and following University of Tennessee Volunteers football, I crisscrossed the state, and continue to, on a regular basis. I began incorporating investigative camping trips into my travels. The first surprise came in West Tennessee at the Civil War site of Fort Pillow State Park. Not only did it offer a view of the Mississippi River from a steep bluff, rivaling any mountain vista, but it proved to be one of the finest campgrounds in this book! Another eye-opener was Nathan Bedford Forrest State Park, a jewel on the Tennessee River, with vistas from on high and a campground where the river lapped my tent site. David Crockett State Park had a fascinating museum. Water was the theme in Middle Tennessee, and I admired the waterfalls at Old Stone Fort and Rock Island state parks. Fall Creek Falls is renowned for its cascades, but new walk-in tent sites sealed it as a premier destination. Water continued to be the theme farther east, where the Obed National Wild and Scenic River has added a high-quality tent campground. In summer I headed for the hills of East Tennessee, where places like Cardens Bluff and high-country campgrounds like Round Mountain kept me cool.

I explored even more campgrounds during the changing seasons and revisited ones I had stayed at before. I recall the spring wildflowers, especially the dwarf crested irises and fire pinks at Land Between The Lakes National Recreation Area; the vistas at Big Hill Pond State Park; the rapids on the Big South Fork; the hot, molasses-slow summer days on Percy Priest Lake; the colorful fall mosaic at North River; and the raw chill at Cosby. With the joy of completing a book and the sadness of an adventure ended, I finished my research. But I continued putting my lessons to work, enjoying more of this underappreciated state, hiking at Nathan Bedford Forrest State Park, fishing Paint Creek, and marveling at the views from atop Frozen Head. I am very grateful and proud to have written this book, and will enjoy my favorite state–Tennessee–for the rest of my life. I hope you will come out and make some Volunteer memories of your own.

–*Johnny Molloy*

# THE BEST
# IN TENT
# CAMPING

## A GUIDE FOR CAR CAMPERS WHO HATE RVs, CONCRETE SLABS, AND LOUD PORTABLE STEREOS

### TENNESSEE

# INTRODUCTION

**T**ENNESSEE IS ONE OF THE OLDEST STATES west of the Appalachian Mountains. Settled by men such as William Blount and James Winchester, the Volunteer State is steeped in American history, from the settlers' gathering to form a state at Sycamore Shoals, to Meriwether Lewis's untimely death on the Natchez Trace, to the Civil War's Fort Pillow. Pioneers traveled on rough overland trails and along rivers used for passage through the vast forests that thrived inland. These high, rich mountains, including the Appalachians and the Cumberland Plateau, still form a rampart to settlement and now offer preserved destinations. Farther west are the floodplains and shores of the Cumberland and Tennessee rivers, with their own unique forests and animal life. The Mississippi River forms the state's western border and has its lowest elevations.

Today tent campers can enjoy these parcels, each a piece of a distinct region of Tennessee. In West Tennessee you can explore the surprisingly hilly terrain of Big Hill Pond on the Mississippi border, or the bluffs and riverine forests of Meeman–Shelby State Park. Middle Tennessee is the land of unique cedar glades, where unusual plants and animals still thrive and where the water falls from the western Cumberland Plateau. This is also lake country, where reservoirs built to prevent disastrous flooding are now recreation destinations, such as Center Hill and Percy Priest Lake. East Tennessee has the highest of the high, including the crest of the Appalachians, where elevations in the Smoky Mountains exceed 6,000 feet. The campgrounds in the Cumberland Mountains offer rock bluffs overlooking gorges cut by water and time, and unique arches and caves.

All this spells paradise for the tent camper. No matter where you go, the scenery will never fail to please. But before embarking on a trip, take time to prepare. Many of the best tent campgrounds are a fair distance from the civilized world, and you want to be enjoying yourself rather than making supply or gear runs. Call ahead and ask for a park map, brochure, or other information to help you plan your trip. Visit the campground's Web site. Make reservations wherever applicable, especially at popular state parks. Ask questions. Ask more questions. The more questions you ask, the fewer surprises you will get. There are other times, however, when you'll grab your gear and this book, hop in the car, and just wing it. This can be an adventure in its own right.

## THE RATING SYSTEM

Included in this book is a rating system for Tennessee's 50 best tent campgrounds. Certain campground attributes—beauty, privacy, spaciousness, quiet, security, and cleanliness—are ranked using a star system. Five stars are ideal; one is acceptable. This system will help you find the campground that has the attributes you desire.

## BEAUTY

In the best campgrounds, the fluid shapes and elements of nature—flora, water, land, and sky—have melded to create locales that seem to have been made for tent camping. The best sites are so attractive you may be tempted not to leave your outdoor home. A little site work is all right to make the scenic area camper-friendly, but too many reminders of civilization eliminated many a campground from inclusion in this book.

## PRIVACY

A little understory goes a long way toward making you comfortable once you've picked your site for the night. There is a trend toward planting natural borders between campsites if the borders don't already exist. With some trees or brush to define the sites, everyone has their personal space, so you can go about the pleasures of tent camping without minding your neighbors.

## SPACIOUSNESS

This attribute can be very important, depending on how much of a gearhead you are and what size your group is. Campers with family-style tents need a large, flat spot on which to pitch their tent, but still need to be able to get to the ice chest to prepare food while not getting burned by the fire ring. Gearheads need adequate space to show all their stuff off to passersby. I just want enough room to keep my bedroom, den, and kitchen separate.

## QUIET

The music of the mountains, rivers, and land between—the singing birds, rushing streams, and wind whooshing through the trees—includes the kinds of noises tent campers associate with being in Tennessee. In concert, they camouflage the sounds you don't want to hear—autos coming and going, loud neighbors, and so on.

## SECURITY

Campground security is relative. A remote campground with no civilization nearby is usually safe, but don't tempt potential thieves by leaving your valuables out for all to see. Use common sense, and go with your instinct. Campground hosts are wonderful to have around, and state parks with locked gates are ideal for security. Get to know your neighbors and, when possible, develop a buddy system for watching each other's belongings.

## CLEANLINESS

I'm a stickler for this one. Nothing will sabotage a scenic campground like trash. Most of the campgrounds in this guidebook are clean. More rustic campgrounds—my favorites—usually receive less maintenance. Busy weekends and holidays will show their effects; however, don't let a little litter spoil your good time. Help clean up, and think of it as doing your part for Tennessee's natural environment.

## HELPFUL HINTS

To make the most of your tent-camping trip, call ahead whenever possible. If going to a state or national park, call for an informative brochure before setting out. This way you can familiarize yourself with the area. Once there, ask questions. Most stewards of the land are proud of their piece of terra firma and are honored you came to visit. They're happy to help you have the best time possible.

If traveling to the Cherokee National Forest, call ahead and order a forest map. Not only will a map make it that much easier to reach your destination, but nearby hikes, scenic drives, waterfalls, and landmarks will be easier to find. There are forest visitor centers in addition to ranger stations. Call or visit and ask questions. When ordering a map, ask for any additional literature about the area in which you are interested.

In writing this book I had the pleasure of meeting many friendly, helpful people: local residents proud of the unique lands around them, and state park and national forest employees who endured my endless questions. Even better were my fellow tent campers, who were eager to share what they knew about their favorite spots. They already know what beauty lies on the horizon. As Tennessee becomes more populated, these lands become that much more precious. Enjoy them, protect them, and use them wisely.

# WEST TENNESSEE

# BIG HILL POND STATE PARK

**B**IG HILL POND STATE PARK is the best-kept secret in West Tennessee. The park was created in part because of its wetlands, which lie in the floodplain of the Tuscumbia River. But this park is not all about wetlands, for Big Hill Pond mostly has steep hills broken by rock outcrops hovering over sharp, wooded ravines. A walk on any of the 30 miles of trails here will testify to that. The entire trail system, with loop possibilities ideal for day hikers, is special enough to have been designated a National Recreation Trail. And when darkness comes, you will find that the campground was seemingly designed with tent campers in mind.

> *This is the most underused and underappreciated state park in West Tennessee.*

The 30-site campground is set on a ridge above Dismal Branch. This rolling backdrop offers vertical variation on your camping opportunities. Enter a classic campground loop shaded by tall pines, hickories, and oaks. Campsites are made level in this hilly country by landscaping timbers. The first few sites are the most open and sunny. Dense woods shade the other campsites. Smaller trees form a thick understory. Campsites are ample in size for the average tent camper and gear. Campsite privacy, while excellent, isn't much of an issue, as this undiscovered getaway is rarely crowded.

As you continue around the loop, a small side road has a few pull-through sites. An intermittent streambed runs along the second half of the loop. There are more dogwoods and pines here. To complete the loop, climb past some sites that are a bit pinched in. There is a fully equipped bathhouse in the center of the loop, along with a couple of campsites. The campground is in the heart of the park which

## RATINGS

Beauty: ☆ ☆ ☆ ☆ ☆
Privacy: ☆ ☆ ☆ ☆ ☆
Spaciousness: ☆ ☆ ☆
Quiet: ☆ ☆ ☆ ☆ ☆
Security: ☆ ☆ ☆ ☆ ☆
Cleanliness: ☆ ☆ ☆ ☆ ☆

## KEY INFORMATION

| | |
|---|---|
| **ADDRESS:** | 11701 Highway 57 Pocahontas, TN 38061 |
| **OPERATED BY:** | Tennessee State Parks |
| **INFORMATION:** | (731) 645-7967; www.tnstateparks. com |
| **OPEN:** | Year-round |
| **SITES:** | 30 |
| **EACH SITE HAS:** | Picnic table, fire ring, upright grill |
| **ASSIGNMENT:** | First come, first served; no reservations |
| **REGISTRATION:** | Ranger will come by to register you |
| **FACILITIES:** | Hot showers, water spigots; bathhouse closed November– February |
| **PARKING:** | At campsites only |
| **FEE:** | $13 per night |
| **ELEVATION:** | 500 feet |
| **RESTRICTIONS:** | Pets: On 6-foot leash only Fires: In fire rings only Alcohol: Prohibited Vehicles: Maximum 2 vehicles per site Other: Maximum 14-day stay |

gives it an honest sense of being in the real, natural Tennessee. Spring and fall are the more popular seasons, but even then Big Hill Pond very rarely fills.

The name Big Hill Pond comes from a dug pond that came to be in 1853 when fill was needed to complete the railroad that runs along the southern side of the park. The cypress-ringed pond is still there. Travis McNatt Lake is a more recent recreational centerpiece. Both lakes offer fishing, but Big Hill Pond is a little harder to access, whereas Travis McNatt Lake is just a short piece from the campground. Spring-fed and 165 acres in size, the lake has lots of bass, bream, and catfish. Even if you don't catch anything, the "no gas motors" lake is a pleasure to paddle in a canoe, especially in spring when the azaleas are blooming, or when autumn's paintbrush reflects off the water.

A 30-mile trail system explores the high and the low of Big Hill Pond State Park and features a little Civil War history, such as the earthworks that were part of a guard post built by Union soldiers to protect the railroad. The highest of the high is an observation tower where there are 360-degree views of the surrounding countryside, including views far south into Mississippi, across the Tuscumbia River Valley. The lowest of the low is the 0.8-mile boardwalk traversing Dismal Swamp, a bottomland forest that attracts waterfowl and other wildlife. In between are wooded hills and surprisingly steep valleys. You may even see deer on the ridges and waterfowl in the lake or hear turkeys gobble in the far distance. The narrow paths meander over clear streams on smaller footbridges and past old homesites where subsistence farmers once eked out a living. These days you will see Mother Nature thriving here in a much richer fashion.

## MAP

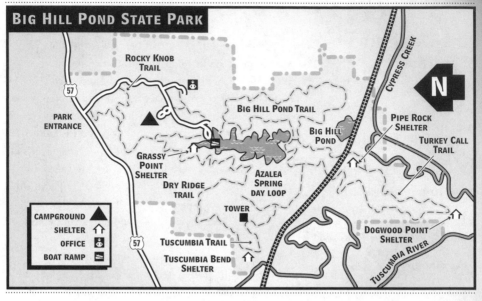

**BIG HILL POND STATE PARK**

ROCKY KNOB TRAIL

PARK ENTRANCE

BIG HILL POND TRAIL

PIPE ROCK SHELTER

BIG HILL POND

TURKEY CALL TRAIL

CYPRESS CREEK

GRASSY POINT SHELTER

DRY RIDGE TRAIL

AZALEA SPRING DAY LOOP

TOWER

DOGWOOD POINT SHELTER

TUSCUMBIA RIVER

| CAMPGROUND | ▲ |
| SHELTER | ⇧ |
| OFFICE | ⬥ |
| BOAT RAMP | ⬗ |

TUSCUMBIA TRAIL

TUSCUMBIA BEND SHELTER

**N**

### GETTING THERE

From Selmer, head 7 miles south on US 45 to TN 57. Turn right and head 10 miles west on TN 57 to the Big Hill Pond entrance, which will be on your left.

# CHICKASAW
# STATE PARK

> *Stay at a lakeside tent camp and enjoy the varied recreational opportunities.*

**C**HICKASAW **STATE PARK** and the surrounding Chickasaw State Forest comprise more than 14,000 acres. Part of the acreage has been developed for intense recreational use, and it is in this segment that the three state park campgrounds lie. Fortunately for us, the tent camp area is located in a picturesque, hilly section along the park's Lake Placid. Lake Placid offers water activities just a short walk from the campground. Horse, hiking, and motor trails spill out from the state park into the adjacent state forest, offering plenty of paths to roam.

A camp store, open in summer, is opposite the trailer camp, which is located hillside in tall pine woods sprinkled with cedars and hardwoods. A thin understory with some grass is offset by decent spacing between campsites. The trailer camp is divided into two loops with bathhouses in the center of each. The pull-ins at many sites are so sloped as to render them nearly unusable by an RV. Tent campers who want electricity will seek these sites. There is a campground host for your safety and convenience.

Wrangler Camp is located below the Lake Placid dam. It is the only campground open year-round. Non-equestrians can use it only in winter, when the other camps are closed. The sites are well spaced and open, with some shade from tall pines and a few cypress trees. Grass carpets the campground floor. Wrangler Camp has its own bathhouse as well.

Lake Placid's tent camp is the preferred destination for this book's readers. It is located on the southern shore of the impoundment fed by Piney Creek. Pine, oak, and hickory trees cover the vertically varied woodland. Sites are widely spread along a ridge-running road leading toward the water. Shady hollows flank the ridgeline. A good mixture of sun and shade allows campers to choose a spot that appeals to their

## RATINGS

Beauty: ☆ ☆ ☆ ☆
Privacy: ☆ ☆ ☆ ☆
Spaciousness: ☆ ☆ ☆
Quiet: ☆ ☆ ☆ ☆
Security: ☆ ☆ ☆ ☆ ☆
Cleanliness: ☆ ☆ ☆ ☆ ☆

preference. Some sites have circular picnic tables. A fully equipped bathhouse stands in the center of an auto turnaround. On the outside of the turnaround are several large, attractive sites that overlook the lake. Landscaping timbers have been used to level the campsites.

A side road spurs off the turnaround and leads down to the lake. Attractive, though smaller, sites with a lake view are spread along both sides of this road. There are a couple sites directly on the lake just before the road dead-ends at a footbridge spanning Lake Placid. There are water spigots throughout the campground.

With Lake Placid so close, why not walk the Lakeshore Nature Trail that runs along the tent camp, or cross the footbridge over to the swimming beach? The clear, cool lake is inviting in summer. High-dive and low-dive boards add a little zing to swimmers' water entrances. Paddleboats and rowboats are available for rent. No private boats are allowed. Many folks choose to wet a line from the bank or a boat, vying for bass and bluegill.

If you want to stay on land, hike the Forked Pine Nature Trail, which leaves from near the picnic shelters. If horseback riding is your thing, an on-site equestrian stable leads trail rides. Beyond the park recreation area, the state forest has more than 50 miles of gravel roads and trails for horse, hikers, mountain bikers, and autos. A forest map is available at the park office. All they ask is that you stay on the established paths and roads.

Chickasaw also has a more-developed side, with tennis, basketball, and volleyball courts; horseshoe pits; an archery range; and playgrounds. Parents will be glad to know that in summer a park recreation director keeps kids busy with arts, crafts, games, movies, and evening programs. The recreational opportunities at Chickasaw run the gamut, so you shouldn't suffer from boredom; just remember to throw in a little relaxation while you're at it.

## KEY INFORMATION

| | |
|---|---|
| **ADDRESS:** | 20 Cabin Lane Henderson, TN 38340 |
| **OPERATED BY:** | Tennessee State Parks |
| **INFORMATION:** | (731) 989-5141; www.tnstateparks. com |
| **OPEN:** | RV and Lake Placid Tent Camp mid-March–November; Wrangler Camp year-round |
| **SITES:** | 121 |
| **EACH SITE HAS:** | Picnic table, lantern post, upright grill, fire ring (Lake Placid Tent Camp); water, electricity, picnic table, upright grills, fire ring (Trailer Camp and Wrangler Camp) |
| **ASSIGNMENT:** | First come, first served; no reservations |
| **REGISTRATION:** | Ranger will come by to register you |
| **FACILITIES:** | Hot showers, water spigots |
| **PARKING:** | At campsites only |
| **FEE:** | Lake Placid Tent Camp $11 per night; Trailer Camp and Wrangler Camp $17 per night |
| **ELEVATION:** | 480 feet |
| **RESTRICTIONS:** | Pets: On 6-foot leash only Fires: In fire rings only Alcohol: Prohibited Vehicles: Maximum 2 vehicles per site Other: Maximum 14-day stay |

**THE BEST IN TENT CAMPING TENNESSEE**

# MAP

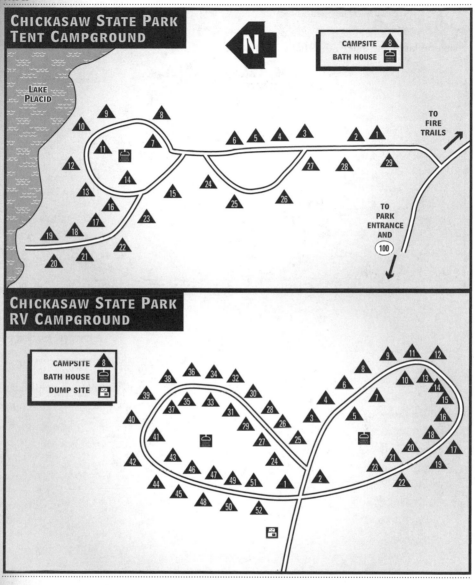

**CHICKASAW STATE PARK TENT CAMPGROUND**

LAKE PLACID

N

CAMPSITE
BATH HOUSE

TO FIRE TRAILS

TO PARK ENTRANCE AND 100

**CHICKASAW STATE PARK RV CAMPGROUND**

CAMPSITE
BATH HOUSE
DUMP SITE

# MAP

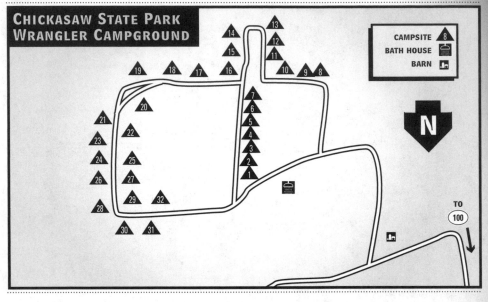

**CHICKASAW STATE PARK**
**WRANGLER CAMPGROUND**

CAMPSITE
BATH HOUSE
BARN

N

TO
100

## GETTING THERE

From Henderson, head west
on TN 100 to the entrance
of Chickasaw State Park,
which will be 10 miles down
on your left.

# FORT PILLOW STATE PARK

> *Fort Pillow has one of the best campgrounds in this entire guidebook.*

**S**IMPLY PUT, I LOVE THIS CAMPGROUND. Why, you ask? It has everything that a tent camper could desire: the sites are in an attractive wooded setting and are well designed; campsite spaciousness and privacy is above average; the camp rarely fills or is even crowded; and there are lots of outdoor activities nearby in which to indulge. Seeing this campground on an ideal Friday evening, I was shocked to find a mere one tent staked out!

Enter the campground, which is divided into three loops. The upper loop occupies the highest spot on a hill. It is heavily wooded, yet is the least wooded of the three loops. Hickory, maple, and oak trees shade the spacious and well-spaced sites. Grass covers much of the loop. The apex of the loop has sites that look out over the Mississippi River through the trees. A fully equipped bathhouse stands in the center of the loop.

The middle loop has more big trees, especially beech, and offers vertical variation among steep, wooded ravines. The loop road winds closely among these trees. Attractive, well-separated campsites lie on the edge of these drop-offs. The hills add to already superlative campsite privacy. Water spigots are adequately spaced here, as they are in the whole campground. The southern loop shows that the situation can get even better. This loop is for tenters only. Many of these sites are walk-in tent sites that afford even more solitude. I recommend this loop above all others, though there is not a bad site in the campground.

Fort Pillow fills only during special events, such as Civil War reenactments. Other than that you can get a site any weekend of the year. The bugs can be troublesome at certain times of the year. Call the park office ahead of time to assess this potential concern.

As with many state parks in the South, Civil War action at this site has led to its being preserved as both

## RATINGS

Beauty: ✪ ✪ ✪ ✪ ✪
Privacy: ✪ ✪ ✪ ✪ ✪
Spaciousness: ✪ ✪ ✪ ✪
Quiet: ✪ ✪ ✪ ✪ ✪
Security: ✪ ✪ ✪ ✪ ✪
Cleanliness: ✪ ✪ ✪ ✪ ✪

a historical and natural area. Located on the Chicka-saw Bluffs overlooking the Mississippi River, the park will impresses you with its natural beauty. The Mighty Mississip' used to run to the edge of the bluffs before the river changed course. The old route of the river is known as the Chute and is an oxbow lake. Back in 1861 the Confederate Army built extensive fortifica-tions here to defend the river. The year 1862 saw a gun battle nearby, and later the Union bombarded Fort Pil-low which ultimately resulted in its being abandoned by the Confederates and occupied by Union forces. In 1864 Nathan Bedford Forrest himself attacked the fort. The Rebels carried the day and Forrest asked for sur-render, but the Feds refused. Subsequently, the Con-federates stormed Fort Pillow, overwhelmed the Union, and won the battle. Afterward, both sides aban-doned the fort. Today you can walk the half-mile trail to the fort, in addition to other major interpretive trails. To better understand the battle, visit the interpretive center, which has a video and displays artifacts and other memorabilia. There are also interpretive pro-grams and special events at the park in summer: visi-tors can learn about a soldier's life and Civil War weapons or go on an owl prowl and nature walks. Spring and fall see a Civil War living history and dis-covery performance, in which folks act out what life was like back then and participate in reenactments. Call the park office for the exact dates.

Two loop trails accommodate campers who want to tour the actual grounds of the area that drew both sides' attention. The inner loop runs 3.8 miles, and the outer loop runs 7.8 miles along earthen fortifications and through surprisingly challenging terrain. In addi-tion, there is the 5-mile, one-way Chickasaw Bluffs Trail, which attracts many backpackers. Less strenuous activities include boating and fishing on 15-acre Fort Pillow Lake, where bass, bream, and crappie await your bait. Other nearby attractions include the home of Alex Haley, the author of *Roots,* in nearby Henning; just south of Fort Pillow is the Lower Hatchie National Wildlife Refuge. No matter what you do, save some time for the campground. It is a good one.

## KEY INFORMATION

| | |
|---|---|
| **ADDRESS:** | 3122 Park Road Henning, TN 37841 |
| **OPERATED BY:** | Tennessee State Parks |
| **INFORMATION:** | (731) 738-5581; www.tnstateparks.com |
| **OPEN:** | Year-round |
| **SITES:** | 40 |
| **EACH SITE HAS:** | Picnic table, fire ring, tent pad |
| **ASSIGNMENT:** | First come, first served; no reservations |
| **REGISTRATION:** | Ranger will come by to register you |
| **FACILITIES:** | Hot showers, flush toilets, water spig-ots, laundry |
| **PARKING:** | At campsites only |
| **FEE:** | $8 per night |
| **ELEVATION:** | 420 feet |
| **RESTRICTIONS:** | Pets: On 6-foot leash only Fires: In fire rings only Alcohol: Prohib-ited Vehicles: None Other: Maximum 14-day stay |

## MAP

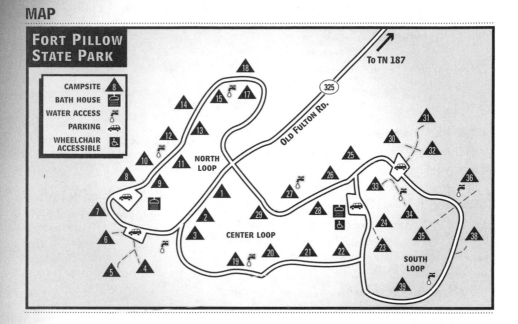

## GETTING THERE

From the junction of TN 54 and US 51 in Covington, head 8.5 miles north on US 51 to TN 87. Turn left onto TN 87 and follow it 17 miles to TN 123, Old Fulton Road. Turn right onto TN 123 and follow it 1 mile to the state park.

# MEEMAN–SHELBY STATE PARK

**T**HE MISSISSIPPI RIVER MADE MEMPHIS. So it is only fitting that a nearby getaway also lies on the banks of the Father of Waters. What surprises visitors are the outdoor opportunities—hiking, biking, and paddling—in this serene park that is *so close* to downtown. (We're talking 15 miles as the crow flies.) Located north of the city on the Chickasaw Bluffs, this park was first developed by the National Park Service and later deeded to the State of Tennessee.

Dogwood Ridge Campground, your base camp, lies beneath a tall deciduous forest of sugar maple, tulip, and sweetgum trees. It is divided into three loops. Smaller trees make for beyond-adequate campsite privacy. The campsites are level, even though the terrain falls away from the campground. Come to the first loop. The first five campsites are the only ones that can be reserved. The spacious sites are spaced well apart from one another. The second loop spurs off the first loop. Younger trees grow among the shade-bearing giants that tower overhead. Pass a fully equipped bathhouse and return to the first loop. Keep passing nice campsites and come to the third loop. This final loop, in a well-groomed, well-cared-for area, is the best. The many dogwood trees here may account for the campground's name. Since there are water and electrical hookups, there will be some big rigs here, but don't let this deter you. Remember, this place was attractive enough for the National Park Service to develop it before deeding it to the State of Tennessee. Meeman–Shelby fills during special events in nearby Memphis and on summer holiday weekends. Other than that you should be able to get a campsite. If you have any worries, just reserve a site.

The vast forests will be the first surprise. Steep-sided ravines drain the Chickasaw Bluffs where large beech, tulip, and sycamore trees grow. Towering oaks

> *This wooded getaway is a world apart from nearby Memphis.*

## RATINGS

Beauty: ☆ ☆ ☆ ☆
Privacy: ☆ ☆ ☆ ☆
Spaciousness: ☆ ☆ ☆ ☆
Quiet: ☆ ☆ ☆ ☆
Security: ☆ ☆ ☆ ☆
Cleanliness: ☆ ☆ ☆ ☆

| | |
|---|---|
| **ADDRESS:** | 910 Riddick Road Millington, TN 38053 |
| **OPERATED BY:** | Tennessee State Parks |
| **INFORMATION:** | (901) 876-5215; www.tnstateparks. com |
| **OPEN:** | Year-round |
| **SITES:** | 49 |
| **EACH SITE HAS:** | Picnic table, fire ring, upright grills, water, electricity |
| **ASSIGNMENT:** | First come, first served; some reservations |
| **REGISTRATION:** | Park visitor center |
| **FACILITIES:** | Hot showers, flush toilets |
| **PARKING:** | At campsites only |
| **FEE:** | $14 per night for tent campers; $16 per night for all others |
| **ELEVATION:** | 350 feet |
| **RESTRICTIONS:** | Pets: On 6-foot leash only Fires: In fire rings only Alcohol: Prohibited Vehicles: None Other: Maximum 14-day stay |

thrive on the higher ground. Giant cottonwoods grow near the river. There are a total of 20 miles of trails to explore; the Chickasaw Trail runs 8 miles along the western edge of Chickasaw Bluffs. Cross the streams flowing to the Mississippi while keeping an eye open for plentiful the wildlife, such as hawks, beavers, and raccoons. The Woodland Trail winds along creeks and past small oxbow lakes in a big forest. Running along the base of the bluffs, the Pioneer Springs Trail passes a historic water source used by both the Chickasaws and original European settlers. Mountain bikers can ply the Bicycle Trail, a 5-mile car-free course. Both paved and gravel roads offer other pedaling opportunities and are often used for biking. Because of the shade cast by tall trees in this 14,000-acre preserve it is a good 10 degrees cooler here in the summer than it is in Memphis.

Sea kayaking has caught up with the Mississippi River. Paddlers drop their boats into the swift water to cruise the scenic shoreline. One trip, requiring a shuttle, heads downstream from Meeman–Shelby 18 miles to Mud Island. Along the way are 100-acre-plus-sized sandbars that make for excellent beachcombing.

As if the mighty Mississippi River isn't water enough for campers, there is also Poplar Tree Lake. Its 125 acres offer anglers bass, bream, and catfish. A fishing pier is available for those without a boat; you can also rent a boat on the spot. If you bring your own boat, remember: only electric motors are allowed, making for a quieter, more pleasant fishing experience. There is a still smaller body of water: a swimming pool open during the summer. Frisbee golf is an unusual pastime enjoyed here. Bring your disc and try your hand on the 18-hole course. There are other outdoor games, too, such as badminton and volleyball. So many choices, so little time—you might have to spend an extra day or two here getting all the fun in.

# MAP

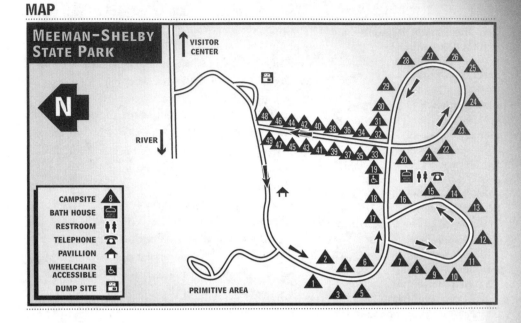

**MEEMAN-SHELBY STATE PARK**

N

VISITOR CENTER

RIVER

| CAMPSITE | 8 |
| BATH HOUSE | |
| RESTROOM | |
| TELEPHONE | |
| PAVILLION | |
| WHEELCHAIR ACCESSIBLE | |
| DUMP SITE | |

PRIMITIVE AREA

## GETTING THERE

From Exit 2-A on I-240 in north Memphis, drive a short distance north to US 51. Head north 4 miles on US 51 to Watkins Road, TN 388. Turn left onto TN 388 and follow it 7 miles to Locke Cuba Road. Turn left onto Locke Cuba Road and follow it 0.5 miles to Bluff Road. Turn right onto Bluff Road to enter the park.

# NATCHEZ TRACE STATE PARK AND FOREST

> *The range of settings and activities is wide enough to suit even tent campers with eclectic tastes.*

**T**HE **NATCHEZ TRACE WAS A TRAVEL** and trade route used by native Indians and settlers. A western branch of this path that once connected Nashville, Tennessee, and Natchez, Mississippi, passed through this park, where today visitors hike, fish, swim, ride horses, and camp on 48,000 acres of attractive forest that was once among the most abused land in the state. Subsequent conservation, begun in the 1930s, has rendered the Natchez an inviting destination. Miles of hiking trails here traverse woodlands, fields, streams, and shorelines. Mountain bikers have miles and miles of backcountry roads and paths to pedal. Park stables offer trail rides, too.

The best destination for tent campers is along Cub Lake. Camping Area 1 runs along a narrow ridgeline toward the lake, and 23 campsites are spread along both sides of the ridge. Landscaping timbers have been used to level the campsites. Overhead is an oak-and-hickory forest with a fairly thick canopy. The sites are well spread apart, though a thin understory lessens campsite privacy. Don't let the fact that these sites have water and electricity make you think this is an RV domain—a new RV campground has been built several miles away in the state park, and all the big rigs head there. Pass the bathhouse and head down to the lake. Just past here are some coveted waterfront sites. At the end of the gravel road are a small play area and a trail leading to the long footbridge crossing Cub Lake.

Camping Area 2 is near the lake but not on it. It has been designated a wilderness camping area. The campsites have not been landscaped or leveled, which gives them a more primitive appearance. There are 44 campsites along two small streams up a hollow. The first few campsites are below the confluence of these small streams and may get extra wet during a major storm. Grass forms the main understory beneath tulip

## RATINGS

Beauty: ✩ ✩ ✩
Privacy: ✩ ✩ ✩
Spaciousness: ✩ ✩ ✩
Quiet: ✩ ✩ ✩ ✩ ✩
Security: ✩ ✩ ✩ ✩
Cleanliness: ✩ ✩ ✩ ✩ ✩

trees, sweetgums, ironwood, dogwoods, and oaks. Come to a fully equipped bathhouse, and the campground road splits. The road to the right heads up the hollow of a small feeder stream. The sites are even hillier here, so be careful where you pitch your tent. The road ends in a teardrop-shaped loop with some widely separated sites.

The other campground road continues up the main hollow and splits left up a dry ridge. There are some sloped sites here, too. Top out by some nice sites, then dip back down into the main hollow. A few sites here have electricity and are also a bit larger than the others. Again, no RVs will dare drive up here. Water spigots are spread throughout the camping area. Beside the RV campground, Pin Oak, there is also a wrangler campground exclusively for folks with horses. Supplies are available at a park store that's open only on weekends.

Recreation is easy to find here. Cub Lake has a swimming beach, and there are rowboats and pedal boats for rent. If you seek the wilder side of Natchez, hit the Cub Creek Trail or the Deer Trail. They are near the campground, too. The Fairview Gullies Trail will give you an idea of how far this area has come since its life as worn-out subsistence farmland a century ago. The Red Leaves Trail makes two loops big enough for overnight backpackers. If you want to ply the woods in greater comfort, take a forest drive. The wildlife area has miles of marked gravel roads, and you can get a map at the park visitor center. Mountain bikers will need this map, too. Horseback trail rides can be arranged at the stables near the wrangler camp.

Want to wet a line? Anglers can visit any of the four lakes that dot the park. Cub Lake is 58 acres and just steps from your tent. Pin Oak Lake, Maple Lake, and Browns Creek Lake all offer angling for crappie, bluegill, bass, and catfish. Rent recreation equipment for activities such as croquet, badminton, and archery. There are many more facilities here, but Natchez is spread out enough to where all park visitors can enjoy the recreation of their choice without its detracting from the natural beauty of the area. Come see for yourself.

## KEY INFORMATION

| | |
|---|---|
| **ADDRESS:** | 24845 Natchez Trace Road Wildersville, TN 38388 |
| **OPERATED BY:** | Tennessee State Parks |
| **INFORMATION:** | (731) 968-3742; www.tnstateparks.com |
| **OPEN:** | Year-round (Camping Area 1); late May–mid-November (Camping Area 2) |
| **SITES:** | 210 |
| **EACH SITE HAS:** | Water, electricity, picnic table, lantern post, upright grill (Camping Area 1); picnic table, lantern post, upright grill, some fire rings (Camping Area 2) |
| **ASSIGNMENT:** | First come, first served; no reservations |
| **REGISTRATION:** | Ranger will come by to register you |
| **FACILITIES:** | Hot showers, water spigots |
| **PARKING:** | At campsites only |
| **FEE:** | $17 per night (Camping Area 1); $1 per night nonelectric, $14 electric (Camping Area 2); $20 per night (Pin Oak) |
| **ELEVATION:** | 400 feet |
| **RESTRICTIONS:** | Pets: On 6-foot leash only Fires: In fire rings only Alcohol: Prohibited Vehicles: None Other: Maximum 14-day stay |

# MAP

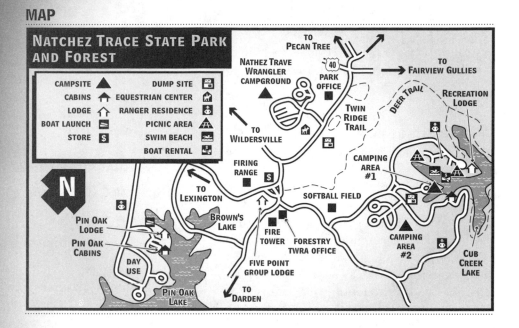

## Natchez Trace State Park and Forest

**Legend:**
- CAMPSITE ▲
- CABINS ♔
- LODGE ⌂
- BOAT LAUNCH
- STORE $
- DUMP SITE
- EQUESTRIAN CENTER
- RANGER RESIDENCE
- PICNIC AREA ⚠
- SWIM BEACH
- BOAT RENTAL

TO PECAN TREE

NATHEZ TRAVE WRANGLER CAMPGROUND

40

PARK OFFICE

TO FAIRVIEW GULLIES

DEER TRAIL

RECREATION LODGE

TWIN RIDGE TRAIL

TO WILDERSVILLE

CAMPING AREA #1

N

TO LEXINGTON

FIRING RANGE

PIN OAK LODGE

PIN OAK CABINS

BROWN'S LAKE

SOFTBALL FIELD

DAY USE

FIRE TOWER

FORESTRY TWRA OFFICE

CAMPING AREA #2

CUB CREEK LAKE

FIVE POINT GROUP LODGE

PIN OAK LAKE

TO DARDEN

## GETTING THERE

From Jackson head east on I-40 to Exit 116. Turn south onto TN 114 and immediately enter the park.

# NATHAN BEDFORD FORREST STATE PARK

**T**HE SITE OF A CIVIL WAR ENGAGEMENT, featuring the highest point in West Tennessee and attractive campsites right on Kentucky Lake, Nathan Bedford Forrest State Park is a land of superlatives. I'll admit it, this place far exceeded my expectations. I drove down to Lakefront Campground first and was happily surprised at the campsites here. Then I went to Pilot Knob, saw the eye-popping view, and learned about this area's place in Tennessee history. The camp's fate was sealed: this state park was definitely to be included in this book.

Let's start with Lakefront Campground. Drive on a dead-end road to come alongside the dammed Tennessee River, now known as Kentucky Lake. You will then find a small, looped road spur with campsites. The sites are large, level squares supported with landscaping timbers. Gravel pads keep the sites well drained. The lake is close enough for you to kick gravel into the water. A low railing keeps campers from falling off the platforms into the water or to the ground below. A tall army of sweetgum trees with a few dogwoods thrown in shades the campsites. A shoreline of small rocks makes entering the water easy. The water spigot is a short walk from the five sites.

Pass the boat ramp and come to the second loop. All the campsites here are lakeside as well. Campsites 10 and 11 share the same extra-large pad, so it can be used as a double site. The loop ends at the thirteenth site. Up the hill is a bathroom with flush toilets; there's a water spigot nearby. At the end of the road are two sites with picnic tables only. These sites are also lakeside.

Happy Hollow Campground is a 38-site affair. It is laid out in a classic loop up a small valley. The first few sites are a bit close together under the tulip, sweetgum, and oak trees. As the loop climbs a small hill, the sites become more open and grassy, appealing to sun

> *The lakeside sites here will lure you back time and again.*

## RATINGS

Beauty: ✩ ✩ ✩ ✩ ✩
Privacy: ✩ ✩ ✩
Spaciousness: ✩ ✩ ✩
Quiet: ✩ ✩ ✩ ✩
Security: ✩ ✩ ✩ ✩
Cleanliness: ✩ ✩ ✩ ✩ ✩

lovers. Some of the sites and the fully equipped bathhouse are in the center of the loop. The sites become more spread out, but a minimal understory keeps campsite privacy about average. Drop back down to a streamside environment for some level, larger, and more attractive sites. There is a campground host here for your convenience.

Anglers and boaters love the proximity of Kentucky Lake to Lakefront Campground: you can almost fish from your tent at some of the sites. There is no designated swimming area, but a whole lake lies before you. However, before you hit the water, consider heading up to Pilot Knob. Catch the view from the point that settlers used as a beacon for many a year. There is an interpretive center up here, too, that focuses on the life and times of those who used to live on the Tennessee River. Admire the memorial to Nathan Bedford Forrest and learn about the Civil War Battle of Johnsonville, where, for the first time in history, a cavalry force defeated a naval force. A ranger conducts programs up here during the warm season. Across the river, Johnsonville State Historic Area offers more insight into the battle and features trails for exploring the now-abandoned town site.

The rugged beauty of the riverside terrain is revealed in the park's trail system, which covers more than 25 miles. Grab a map at the park office. Swing along Pilot Knob Ridge and drop down into hollows that lead to the river's edge. Or just cruise right along the river. Either way, you will appreciate the riverside beauty of this high-quality state park.

## MAP

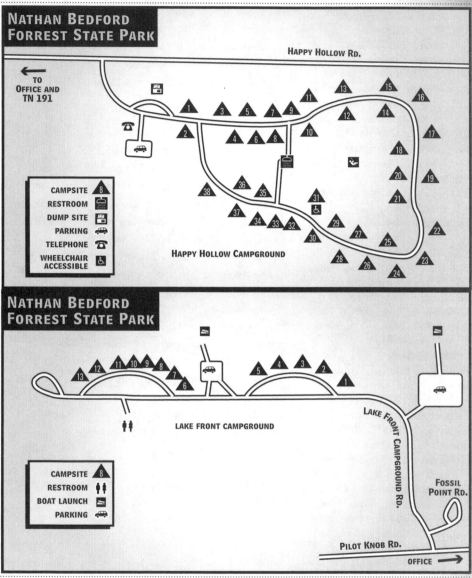

**NATHAN BEDFORD FOREST STATE PARK**

HAPPY HOLLOW RD.

← TO OFFICE AND TN 191

CAMPSITE
RESTROOM
DUMP SITE
PARKING
TELEPHONE
WHEELCHAIR ACCESSIBLE

HAPPY HOLLOW CAMPGROUND

**NATHAN BEDFORD FOREST STATE PARK**

LAKE FRONT CAMPGROUND

CAMPSITE
RESTROOM
BOAT LAUNCH
PARKING

LAKE FRONT CAMPGROUND RD.

FOSSIL POINT RD.

PILOT KNOB RD.

OFFICE →

## GETTING THERE

From the courthouse square in Camden, take TN 191 north 8 miles to the state park.

# PICKWICK LANDING STATE PARK

*Camp at Bruton Branch Recreation Area and tour Shiloh Battlefield while you are here.*

**P**ICKWICK **LANDING STATE PARK** has a dizzying array of offerings, many of which don't necessarily appeal to tent campers, like a lodge and golf course. However, it also has things that do lure in our kind, like Bruton Branch Recreation Area, with a 75-site tent campground overlooking Pickwick Lake. Recreation here is, not surprisingly, water-based. Bruton Branch stands alone, a 350-acre parcel of land across the river from the rest of the state park, which has the lodge and another, more-developed campground. Just outside the park is one of the most notorious battlefields in the United States, Shiloh. I certainly felt it worthwhile to spend a day absorbing the history of this major Civil War conflict. Come to Pickwick, stay at Bruton Branch, and tour Shiloh National Military Park while you are here.

In all fairness, tent campers need to hear about the main campground. The electric and water hookups spell RV, but many of the paved pull-ins are so sloped that no self-respecting big-rig drivers would park there, unless they like sleeping on a hill. However, leveled camping areas mean that tent campers can enjoy this area. The wooded campground is spread out in a series of small, interconnected loops beneath thick hickory, oak, and pine woods. The campsites are well spaced, separated by trees, and served by fully equipped bathhouses.

Across the river lies Bruton Branch Recreation Area. Area 1 is in a cove of the lake. The sites are wooded with a grassy understory and are well spaced, but a lack of understory minimizes campsite privacy. The sites do have good lake views, though. In fact, many of the sites are immediately beside the lake. Area 1 and Area 2 have 13 sites altogether. Continue down Bruton Branch Road and pass a few day-use areas. The next campsites are at Area 5 through Area 8. The cove

## RATINGS

Beauty: ✫ ✫ ✫ ✫
Privacy: ✫ ✫ ✫
Spaciousness: ✫ ✫ ✫
Quiet: ✫ ✫ ✫
Security: ✫ ✫ ✫ ✫
Cleanliness: ✫ ✫ ✫ ✫

has now given way to the main lake, and the lakeside sites have far-reaching views down to Pickwick Dam and across the main park's lake. Past Area 5 the campground begins to widen, and there are sites away from the lake as well as on it. Young hardwoods shade most of the sites.

A swimming beach and boat landing break up the camping area. Farther down, the campground widens into three rows of campsites. All the sites have a view of the lake, but the sites immediately on the lake of course offer the best views and water access. A fully equipped bathhouse stands beside a small ranger station. There is a water spigot here, too. The campground narrows again beyond the bathhouse then ends where Bruton Branch Road dead-ends.

Swimming, fishing, and boating are the top activities at Bruton Branch. The lake dominates the scenery and action. Across the lake, at the park, water recreation is also the name of the game, and you can rent boats at the marina there. There are two more swimming beaches if you want a change of scenery. Also at the main park are volleyball, badminton, and other field games. There is a hiking trail as well, but if you want to walk around I suggest you make the short drive to Shiloh National Military Park.

First go to the Shiloh visitor center to look around and maybe take in the video presentation. Cars or bikes can take the historical-tour route. Pull over and walk around to see the sights here. You will gain real insight into the Civil War, learning about the strategies undertaken by General Ulysses S. Grant and Albert Sidney Johnston, the highest-ranking American officer ever killed in battle, and how the Union vessels on the nearby Tennessee River influenced the outcome of this two-day clash. See the memorials to the soldiers of various states who fought here, then visit the infamous Bloody Pond and learn how Shiloh was the first place where military field hospitals were used. Beyond the main tour route, historic old roads and trails invite further exploration. The history of Shiloh will help you appreciate the pleasantness of your life as you enjoy Bruton Branch.

## KEY INFORMATION

**ADDRESS:** P.O. Box 15 Pickwick Dam, TN 38365

**OPERATED BY:** Tennessee State Parks

**INFORMATION:** (731) 689-3129; www.tnstateparks.com

**OPEN:** Bruton Branch mid-March–mid-October; Main Campground year-round

**SITES:** 123

**EACH SITE HAS:** Picnic table, fire ring (Bruton Branch); water, electricity, picnic tables, upright grill, fire ring (Main Campground)

**ASSIGNMENT:** First come, first served; no reservations

**REGISTRATION:** Ranger will come by to register you

**FACILITIES:** Hot showers, water spigots, pay phone, ice machine

**PARKING:** At campsites only

**FEE:** Bruton Branch $10 per night; Main Campground $15.50 per night for tents, $17.50 per night for RVs

**ELEVATION:** 420 feet

**RESTRICTIONS:** Pets: On 6-foot leash only
Fires: In fire rings only
Alcohol: Prohibited
Vehicles: Maximum 2 vehicles per site
Other: Maximum 14-day stay

## MAP

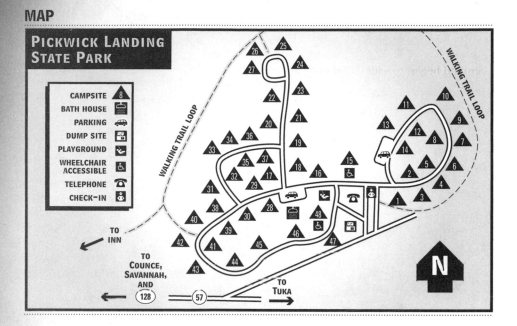

**PICKWICK LANDING STATE PARK**

CAMPSITE

BATH HOUSE

PARKING

DUMP SITE

PLAYGROUND

WHEELCHAIR ACCESSIBLE

TELEPHONE

CHECK-IN

WALKING TRAIL LOOP

WALKING TRAIL LOOP

TO INN

TO COUNCE, SAVANNAH, AND 128

57

TO TUKA

N

## GETTING THERE

From the junction with US 64 in Savannah, head 9.8 miles south on TN 128 to Worley Road. Turn left onto Worley Road and follow it 0.5 miles to Pyburns Drive. Turn right onto Pyburns Drive and follow it 5 miles to Bruton Road. Turn right onto Bruton Road and follow it 0.5 miles to Bruton Branch Road. Veer right onto Bruton Branch Road and follow it to a dead end at the recreation area. The main campground is down TN 128 just beyond Pickwick Dam.

MIDDLE TENNESSEE

# ANDERSON ROAD

**P**ART OF THE ARMY CORPS OF ENGINEER'S Anderson Road Recreation Area, Anderson Road Campground is a wooded oasis in the fast-growing area near Percy Priest Lake. Not only is it a refuge, it is a darn good one, especially for tent campers! These lakefront sites, built by the Army Corps of Engineers, are in great shape but don't have electricity. This keeps out the RVs and leaves the beautiful cedar-wooded peninsula for us alone.

The campground is laid out in a classic loop on land that gently descends toward Percy Priest Lake. The campground host mans the guard station. As soon as you enter the campsite you encounter high-quality lakefront sites. The sites are far from the road and one another and are close to the lake—all the qualities you want in a campsite. Hickory, oak, and walnut trees complement the beautiful evergreen cedar trees. There is some grass in clear places, but the ground is very rocky and full of the crumbly limestone for which this area is known. Some sites are partly open, but there is always adequate shade, and each site has more than adequate privacy. Many of the lakefront sites either look out on the water or have a short path that leads to Percy Priest Lake.

You will undoubtedly notice the unusual, round, concrete picnic tables. You will also notice that the campsites on the inside of the loop, some of which are wonderfully shaded by dense cedar copses, are good, despite being less popular than those on the lakefront. Since campsites can be reserved, you will be able to get a lakefront site if you desire, but the ones away from the lake are better than those at most campgrounds anywhere.

Pass the campground boat ramp for more good campsites. The loop begins to turn away from the lake

> *These are some of my favorite lakefront tent sites in the state.*

## RATINGS

Beauty: ✩ ✩ ✩ ✩ ✩
Privacy: ✩ ✩ ✩
Spaciousness: ✩ ✩ ✩
Quiet: ✩ ✩ ✩
Security: ✩ ✩ ✩ ✩
Cleanliness: ✩ ✩ ✩ ✩

## KEY INFORMATION

**ADDRESS:** 3737 Bell Road
Nashville, TN
37214

**OPERATED BY:** Army Corps of
Engineers

**INFORMATION:** (615) 889-1975;
www.lrn.usace.arm
y.mil; reservations
(877) 444-6777;
www.reserveusa.
com

**OPEN:** Mid-May–early
September

**SITES:** 37

**EACH SITE HAS:** Picnic table, fire
ring, upright grill

**ASSIGNMENT:** First come, first
served, and by
reservation

**REGISTRATION:** At campground
entrance station

**FACILITIES:** Hot showers, flush
toilets, water spig-
ots, laundry

**PARKING:** At campsites only

**FEE:** $12 per night non-
waterfront sites,
$14 per night
waterfront sites

**ELEVATION:** 500 feet

**RESTRICTIONS:** Pets: On leash only
Fires: In fire rings
only
Alcohol: At camp-
sites only
Vehicles: Some
sites allow up to 3
vehicles
Other: Maximum
14-day stay in a
30-day period

at campsite 24, and the road climbs up to pure-woodland campsites that offer maximum privacy. Reach a high point to find more-dispersed sites. I would stay up here to enjoy the easy lake access, but I sometimes get tired of boat noises. Two bathhouses serve the camp. Anderson Road is often full, and reservations are highly recommended.

The 1.3-mile Fitness Trail is part of the Anderson Road Recreation Area complex. The name Fitness Trail implies something more than it is. The path doesn't have exercise stations or any other man-made contraptions. It is merely an easy trail that wanders through cedar woods and glades, offering fantastic lake views as it skirts the shores of Percy Priest Lake. The last portion of the trail turns away from the lake and heads toward a road that is part of the recreation area. You have to walk a bit of the road to complete the loop.

The recreation area also has a swimming beach that is popular with campers and day visitors. You will notice on the way in that the place gets a lot of day use; there are many people living in the immediate area. Percy Priest is an impressive lake. From Anderson Road you can easily see the seemingly low-slung, and long, Percy Priest Dam to the north. The dam is 130 feet high, more than a half-mile long, and 7 miles above the confluence of the Stones and Cumberland rivers. The reservoir drains 865 square miles of the Tennessee landscape. The primary river drainages are East Fork Stones River and West Fork Stones River. Percy Priest Lake is 42 miles long and has 213 miles of curving shoreline. The lake's average depth is 29 feet. The lake project was initiated after World War II as part of the Flood Control Act of 1946. The resultant body of water was originally called Stewarts Ferry Reservoir, but the name was changed to honor the Tennessee congressman J. Percy Priest. Dam construction began in 1963 and took five years to complete. The purpose of the lake is to control flooding on the Cumberland River, generate hydropower, and provide public recreation—and Anderson Road Campground is a high-quality part of that public recreation.

# MAP

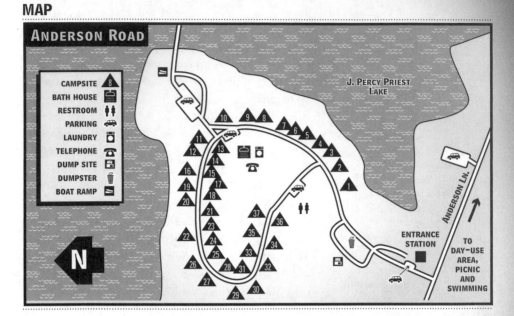

## ANDERSON ROAD

**CAMPSITE** ▲ 8
**BATH HOUSE**
**RESTROOM** ♀♂
**PARKING**
**LAUNDRY**
**TELEPHONE** ☎
**DUMP SITE**
**DUMPSTER**
**BOAT RAMP**

J. PERCY PRIEST LAKE

ANDERSON LN.

ENTRANCE STATION

TO DAY–USE AREA, PICNIC AND SWIMMING

N

## GETTING THERE

From Exit 219 on I-40 east of downtown Nashville take Stewarts Ferry Pike/Bell Road south 4.7 miles to Smith Springs Road. (Soon after leaving the interstate, Stewarts Ferry Pike becomes Bell Road.) Turn left onto Smith Springs Road and follow it 1.1 miles to Anderson Road. Turn left onto Anderson Road and follow it 1.3 miles. The campground is on the left before you reach the primary Anderson Road Recreation Area.

# BLEDSOE CREEK STATE PARK

*Bledsoe Creek makes for a quick getaway from Nashville and is located near interesting historical sites.*

**B**LEDSOE **C**REEK **IS A WOODED REFUGE** from the ever-escalating pace of life in Nashville. Two hundred years ago life was far different. You can explore this history while enjoying the watery recreation of this state park, set on the shores of Old Hickory Lake. The campground is a real hit-and-miss affair, a hodgepodge of good and not-so-good campsites. I recommend inspecting the entire campground before picking your site. The campground fills only on summer holiday weekends, but get here early on other weekends so you can get one of the better sites.

The campground is situated on a hilly peninsula, surrounded on three sides by Old Hickory Lake. Enter the campground and come to Deer Run Road. This section of the campground, which swings around toward the lake, is open year-round. These campsites have paved pull-ins and have little level ground for a tent. There are several lakeside sites that are larger. There is a dock at the end of the road. The understory is mostly grassy with some brush.

Woodchuck Hollow is the next campground road. Many campsites there have circular picnic tables. There is a real mixture of sun and shade, and there is some vegetation between the campsites. Oak and cedar are the dominant trees. The latter half of the loop has large sites. This road, like the others, has a bathhouse.

Blue Heron Drive has the best sites in the park: they are large, heavily shaded, and lakefront. The best of the best are on the auto turnaround at the end of the loop, and these sites will go first. Some sites are pull-up, others pull-through.

Rabbit Jump Hill has widely separated sites, some of which are shady. What makes this section unusual is the pond at the center of the auto turnaround. Sites 103–114, found along Main Park Road, do not have

## RATINGS

Beauty: ✿ ✿ ✿
Privacy: ✿ ✿ ✿ ✿
Spaciousness: ✿ ✿ ✿ ✿
Quiet: ✿ ✿ ✿
Security: ✿ ✿ ✿ ✿ ✿
Cleanliness: ✿ ✿ ✿ ✿ ✿

water or electricity and are favored by tent campers. Some are good, but some are too sloped for a comfortable night's sleep. Be discriminating when you pick a site here.

Once you have made your selection, hit the water or hit the trails. A ramp at the campground makes it easy to launch a boat. Fish Old Hickory, or ski. Most anglers go for the crappie, bluegill, bass, and catfish. You can also fish from the campground's dock.

This state park is managed as an environmental education area. Your ticket to learning about the state park is the 6 miles of trails that are reachable directly from your tent. Check out the lake from along the Shoreline Trail, then get the view from above on the High Ridge Trail. The two trails make for a good loop hike. There are shorter trails, too, including the Birdsong Interpretive Nature Trail.

I have most enjoyed learning about the area's history. Just up the road is Cragfont, the preserved home of General James Winchester, a hero in both the Revolutionary War and the War of 1812. Cragfont, completed in 1802, features impressive stone- and woodwork. You can enjoy views of the garden and the surrounding area from Cragfont, because it is high on a bluff. Not far from here is Wynnewood, a two-story log inn set near mineral springs that attracted buffalo in the days before the United States was a country. Wynnewood was built by A. R. Wynne to be a stage-coach stopover and a getaway for people wishing to enjoy the springs. A National Historic Landmark, the inn survived the Civil War and is furnished with period furniture. Wynnewood is east of the state park on TN 25. To the west of the park, in Hendersonville, is Rock Castle, the home of the Revolutionary War officer Daniel Smith. His house was built with limestone and wood found on his own land. For detailed information on these historic sites, contact the park office.

## KEY INFORMATION

| | |
|---|---|
| **ADDRESS:** | 400 Zieglers Fort Road Gallatin, TN 37066 |
| **OPERATED BY:** | Tennessee State Parks |
| **INFORMATION:** | (615) 452-3706; www.tnstateparks.com |
| **OPEN:** | Deer Run open year-round; rest of campground mid-April–November |
| **SITES:** | 114 |
| **EACH SITE HAS:** | Picnic table, rock fire ring; most have water and electricity |
| **ASSIGNMENT:** | First come, first served; no reservations |
| **REGISTRATION:** | Self-registration on-site |
| **FACILITIES:** | Hot showers, flush toilets, pay phone, laundry |
| **PARKING:** | At campsites only |
| **FEE:** | $12 per night tent sites, $18 per night other sites |
| **ELEVATION:** | 500 feet |
| **RESTRICTIONS:** | Pets: On 6-foot leash only<br>Fires: In fire rings only<br>Alcohol: Not allowed<br>Vehicles: None<br>Other: 14-day stay limit |

## MAP

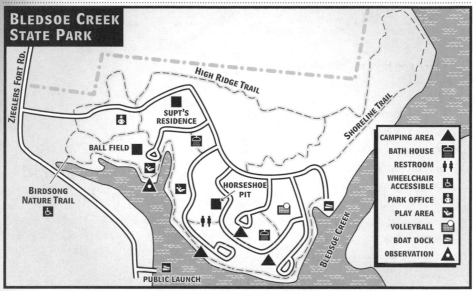

**BLEDSOE CREEK STATE PARK**

ZIEGLERS FORT RD.

HIGH RIDGE TRAIL

SHORELINE TRAIL

SUPT'S RESIDENCE

BALL FIELD

BIRDSONG NATURE TRAIL

HORSESHOE PIT

BLEDSOE CREEK

PUBLIC LAUNCH

| | |
|---|---|
| CAMPING AREA | |
| BATH HOUSE | |
| RESTROOM | |
| WHEELCHAIR ACCESSIBLE | |
| PARK OFFICE | |
| PLAY AREA | |
| VOLLEYBALL | |
| BOAT DOCK | |
| OBSERVATION | |

## GETTING THERE

From downtown Gallatin, head 5 miles east TN 25 to Zieglers Fort Road. Turn right onto Zieglers Fort Road and follow it 1.8 miles to the park entrance, on the left.

# CEDARS OF LEBANON STATE PARK

**C**EDARS OF **L**EBANON **S**TATE **P**ARK doubles as a recreation getaway and a preserve for a unique remnant of cedar forest, native to Tennessee. The forest is America's largest remaining woodland of its type. As nearby Nashville grows, these 9,000 acres will become even more valuable. Tent campers will appreciate the campground, which has a loop that allows tents, pop-ups, and vans only; RV campers have their own area. Developed recreation, such as a pool and game courts, lies near the campground. Campers can also explore the cedar forests that caused this area to be preserved in the first place.

> *This state park has America's largest remaining cedar forest and more.*

The first area, Campground 1, is laid out like a parking lot, with pull-through sites and way too much pavement. It is RV headquarters, so don't even bother. Campground 2 is much more heavily wooded and has a lot less pavement. There are campsites on both sides of the loop, which has a little vertical variation and some hardwood trees. Some sites are a bit close together but will do. Gravel pads ringed by landscaping timbers make the sites more conducive to tent camping. Campground 3, which is the largest but has the fewest campsites, is the best because it offers more privacy and space. Grass and brush form the understory of a forest that thickens beyond the first few campsites. The paved pull-ins do not diminish the atmosphere here. The campsites in the back half of the loop are very spread apart and are raised a bit because heavy rains can inundate the woods near the loop. An intermittent streambed runs along the far end of the loop. The last few sites are open and sunny and are preferable on cooler days.

## RATINGS

Beauty: ☆ ☆ ☆ ☆
Privacy: ☆ ☆ ☆ ☆
Spaciousness: ☆ ☆ ☆
Quiet: ☆ ☆ ☆
Security: ☆ ☆ ☆ ☆
Cleanliness: ☆ ☆ ☆ ☆

## KEY INFORMATION

| | |
|---|---|
| **ADDRESS:** | 328 Cedar Forest Road<br>Lebanon, TN 37090 |
| **OPERATED BY:** | Tennessee State Parks |
| **INFORMATION:** | (615) 443-2769;<br>www.tnstateparks.com |
| **OPEN:** | Year-round |
| **SITES:** | 117 |
| **EACH SITE HAS:** | Picnic table, fire ring, water, electricity, lantern post, upright grill |
| **ASSIGNMENT:** | First come, first served; no reservations |
| **REGISTRATION:** | At camp store in summer; ranger will come by in winter |
| **FACILITIES:** | Hot showers, flush toilets, pay phone |
| **PARKING:** | At campsites only |
| **FEE:** | Tents $14 per night, RVs $17 per night |
| **ELEVATION:** | 700 feet |
| **RESTRICTIONS:** | Pets: On 6-foot leash only<br>Fires: In fire rings only<br>Alcohol: Prohibited<br>Vehicles: None<br>Other: Maximum 14-day stay |

A camp store and laundry, open during the warm season, is accessible to all campers. Campsites at Cedars of Lebanon do not fill up except on summer holiday weekends. There are many recreation facilities at this park, including an ultralarge swimming pool just a short walk from the campground, and a disc golf course. You can purchase a disc at the camp store. The swimming pool is open from Memorial Day to Labor Day. Game courts are another option—there are volleyball and tennis courts and horseshoe pits. The park's nature center is open during the summer; here you can learn more about the unique cedar forest and also take advantage of ranger-led programs: kids and adults alike will enjoy learning about insects and snakes and how nature works. The rangers will also tell you about the area's cedar glades, natural clearings in the forest that host such plants as cactus and reindeer moss and other living things unusual for this region. Also learn about the cedar trees, for which the park is named; cedars were also used by early settlers to build cabins and fences and make roof shingles. The wood was preferred because it splits easily and is rot-resistant. In later years the cedar forests were commercially logged, with their wood used primarily to make pencils because it is light and easily sharpened. Today the cedar forest has made a comeback to stretch along the 8 miles of park trails that wind through the evergreens. Shorter nature trails, such as the Limestone Sinks Trail and the Hidden Springs Trail, are good leg-stretcher walks near the campground. If you don't feel like walking, go horseback riding. A park stable offers guided rides through the Middle Tennessee woods along miles of bridle paths.

# MAP

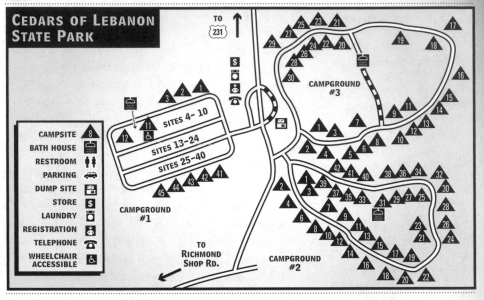

**CEDARS OF LEBANON STATE PARK**

TO 231

Legend:
- CAMPSITE 8
- BATH HOUSE
- RESTROOM
- PARKING
- DUMP SITE
- STORE $
- LAUNDRY
- REGISTRATION
- TELEPHONE
- WHEELCHAIR ACCESSIBLE

SITES 4-10
SITES 13-24
SITES 25-40

CAMPGROUND #1

CAMPGROUND #2

CAMPGROUND #3

TO RICHMOND SHOP RD.

## GETTING THERE

From Exit 238 on I-40 near Lebanon, head 6 miles south on US 231 to the state park entrance, which will be on your left.

# DAVID CROCKETT
# STATE PARK

*This area offers plenty of activities both inside and outside the park.*

IT SEEMS THAT FEW OF DAVID CROCKETT'S real-life adventures and accomplishments overshadow the "myths" imparted by the Disney television show of the early 1960s about our Tennessee hero. The primary myth is that he was called "Davy" Crockett. In fact, he went by David, and Mr. Crockett may well have been put off by being called Davy. That was just one of the many things I learned while visiting the museum at this park that also offers outdoor recreation and some pretty decent tent camping.

Crystal-clear Shoal Creek is the centerpiece of the park. It was along this creek that Crockett had a gristmill, a powder mill, and a distillery. Where you camp at this park has seen a lot of changes through the years. A flood in 1821 washed away Crockett's creekside "empire," and he left for West Tennessee. Nowadays, Shoal Creek flows through the park and borders the main camping area, Campground 1. There are scattered trees, but much of the understory is grassy. Campground 1 is the best for tent campers. The main road curves toward Shoal Creek then comes to the preferred sites, starting with 15. The preferred sites back up to the pretty waterway and extend through site 30. The main camping area then turns away from the creek. However, the unnumbered primitive overflow camping area continues along Shoal Creek. Its sites are the best of the best, though they are the most rustic. They do feature a bathhouse and covered picnic shelter however. The rolling hills, grassy areas, and creek make this the better camping area for those with kids.

Campground 2 is deeper into the park and atop a ridgeline. The sites, all with water and electricity, are smaller and more crammed together and slope off a steep hillside. Tent campers will have a tough time finding a level site up here, as most of the campers are sleeping in rigs that are on campsite parking pads.

## RATINGS

Beauty: ☆ ☆ ☆
Privacy: ☆ ☆ ☆
Spaciousness: ☆ ☆ ☆
Quiet: ☆ ☆ ☆
Security: ☆ ☆ ☆ ☆ ☆
Cleanliness: ☆ ☆ ☆ ☆

Each campsite does have unusual elevated fire rings—metal cylinders stuck in the ground. Most campers that come to this park return again and again. These campgrounds are full some summer weekends, especially during David Crockett Days in mid-August. Other than that you should be able to get a site.

I like the wide variety of activities available both inside and outside the park. Developed park facilities include an Olympic-sized swimming pool and a park restaurant that overlooks 40-acre Lake Lindsey where anglers can catch bass, bream, and catfish. If you don't want to fish from shore, rent a park paddleboat or johnboat. Private boats and motors are not allowed, which makes for a quiet and rustic experience. I particularly enjoyed the park museum, which, of course, features exhibits on David Crockett and describes what life was once like in this part of the Volunteer State. Don't pass this up! If you want to learn still more, attend one of the park's interpretive programs, which range from musical shows to exhibits of 18th-century clothing and the owls of Tennessee. You can even learn how to throw a tomahawk!

Traditional outdoor pursuits include hiking on the park trails. My favorite trail is the one along Shoal Creek. This stream is so clear I couldn't get enough of looking at it! Speaking of Shoal Creek, you can fish it too: trout are stocked here in the spring.

Many people like to head into town, which is only 2 miles away, or eat in the park restaurant. History buffs will want to check out the James D. Vaughan and David Crockett museums in Lawrenceburg. Crockett is worth two museums of history and maybe more. Farther afield are the Amish farms, where campers can take wagon and buggy tours of the Amish country adjacent to Lawrenceburg. This experience will round out your "Crockett country" adventure. Just remember, it's David Crockett, not Davy.

## KEY INFORMATION

| | |
|---|---|
| **ADDRESS:** | 1400 West Gaines Lawrenceburg, TN 38464 |
| **OPERATED BY:** | Tennessee State Parks |
| **INFORMATION:** | (615) 532-0001; www.tnstateparks.com |
| **OPEN:** | Year-round |
| **SITES:** | 108 |
| **EACH SITE HAS:** | Picnic table, fire ring; most also have water and electricity |
| **ASSIGNMENT:** | First come, first served, no reservations |
| **REGISTRATION:** | At park office |
| **FACILITIES:** | Hot showers, flush toilets, ice machine |
| **PARKING:** | At campsites only |
| **FEE:** | $15.50 per night electric sites, $8 per night primitive sites |
| **ELEVATION:** | 800 feet |
| **RESTRICTIONS:** | Pets: On leash only Fires: In fire rings only Alcohol: Prohibited Vehicles: Maximum 2 vehicles per site Other: Maximum 2 tents per site |

# MAP

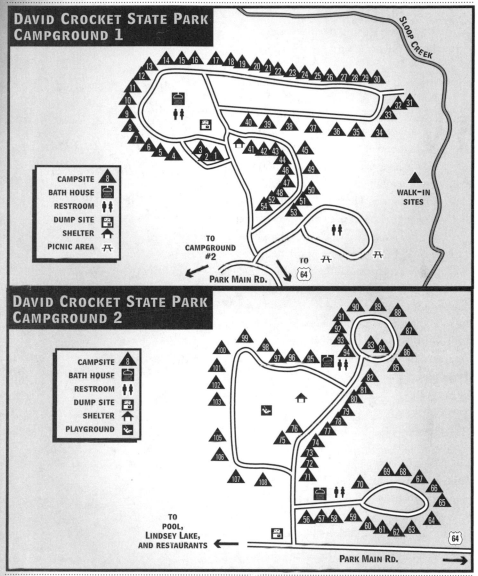

**DAVID CROCKET STATE PARK CAMPGROUND 1**

| | |
|---|---|
| CAMPSITE | 8 |
| BATH HOUSE | |
| RESTROOM | |
| DUMP SITE | |
| SHELTER | |
| PICNIC AREA | |

WALK-IN SITES

TO CAMPGROUND #2

TO 64

PARK MAIN RD.

SLOOP CREEK

**DAVID CROCKET STATE PARK CAMPGROUND 2**

| | |
|---|---|
| CAMPSITE | 8 |
| BATH HOUSE | |
| RESTROOM | |
| DUMP SITE | |
| SHELTER | |
| PLAYGROUND | |

TO POOL, LINDSEY LAKE, AND RESTAURANTS

PARK MAIN RD.

64

## GETTING THERE

From the junction of US 64 and TN 43 in Lawrenceburg, take US 64 west 1 mile to the state park, on your right.

# EDGAR EVINS
# STATE PARK

**W**HILE **I** WAS TOURING THE STATE in search of the best campsites around, the campground at Edgar Evins State Park caught my attention. This park is set on the shores of Center Hill Lake, where innumerable steep, folded hills offer outstanding scenery. There is very little flat land, and this forced campground designers to construct some very unusual campsites, which ended up being the most unusual, by far, of those in the book you are reading. When glancing at the accompanying campground map, you will see that Edgar Evins State Park's campground looks like a mere series of loops. What the map does not show is the extremely steep terrain from which large, level, wooden camping platforms supported by concrete and metal poles extend from the sloping terrain. So, you literally pitch your tent on a level platform notwithstanding that the ground recedes below you. The picnic tables are on the platform, but the upright grill and fire rings are on the land, by the platform. No smart camper would want to have his or her fire ring or grill on a wooden platform! This platform setup literally has campers hanging out in the trees. Low wooden fences border the platforms to keep you from falling off them. The experience is akin to camping on a deck looking out on the land below. And I like it.

The campground as a whole is set on a large slope leading down to Center Hill Lake. Campsites 1 through 12 are on the highest road and are farthest from the water; therefore, they're the least used. But I recommend them for solitude. The middle area, with sites 13 through 34, is the least desirable. It is neither

> *The platform campsites here are most unusual.*

## RATINGS

Beauty: ✩ ✩ ✩
Privacy: ✩ ✩ ✩
Spaciousness: ✩ ✩ ✩
Quiet: ✩ ✩ ✩ ✩
Security: ✩ ✩ ✩ ✩ ✩
Cleanliness: ✩ ✩ ✩ ✩

| | |
|---|---|
| **ADDRESS:** | 1630 Edgar Evins Park Road Silver Point, TN 38582 |
| **OPERATED BY:** | Tennessee State Parks |
| **INFORMATION:** | (931) 858-2446; www.tnstateparks.com |
| **OPEN:** | Year-round |
| **SITES:** | 60 |
| **EACH SITE HAS:** | Picnic table, fire ring, upright grill, water, electricity |
| **ASSIGNMENT:** | First come, first served; no reservations |
| **REGISTRATION:** | At registration building |
| **FACILITIES:** | Hot showers, flush toilets, laundry |
| **PARKING:** | At campsites only |
| **FEE:** | $18 per night |
| **ELEVATION:** | 750 feet |
| **RESTRICTIONS:** | Pets: On leash only Fires: In fire rings only Alcohol: Prohibited Vehicles: None Other: Maximum 14-day stay |

high nor by the water. The third group of sites, 35 through 60, is very nice. These sites are all on the outside of the loop and extend out toward the water. Informal trails lead from the campsites to the steep edge of the lake. Starting with 43, the sites are designated waterfront. And here at Edgar Evins State Park, campers are not charged extra for a waterfront site! As an added bonus, campsites 35 through 60 are open year-round, for cold-weather excursions.

But Edgar Evins State Park is primarily a warm-weather summertime destination that fills on summer holiday weekends. Lots of tent campers use this park to enjoy water-based recreation on Center Hill Lake. The park has two boat launches, a boat dock, and a marina. The marina rents boats and has a small store. There is no designated swim area—campers swim at their own risk on the lake. The state park is on Center Hill Lake, but it is also near the below-dam outflow of the Caney Fork River, which is great for canoeing and fishing. Outfitters are conveniently located at the state park entrance. They will rent a canoe and shuttle you for a fee. Make the time to enjoy this riverine parcel of the Volunteer State.

There are also land-based activities at Edgar Evins. The park office loans out any number of recreational items, such as badminton equipment. But you ought to enjoy the natural side of this state park, for it has one of the best hiking trails in Middle Tennessee, the Millennium Trail. Laid out by the Tennessee Trails Association, the trail takes you on a rugged, challenging hike through formerly settled land, across rocky ridges, along lakeside bluffs, and through lush wooded hollows. This is a challenging hike, no doubt about it, so have your game face on. The Highland Rim Nature Trail is shorter, at 2.4 miles, but it also has some steep ups and downs. But that is no surprise for a place where the campground had to have wooden platforms erected just to have some level land to camp!

# MAP

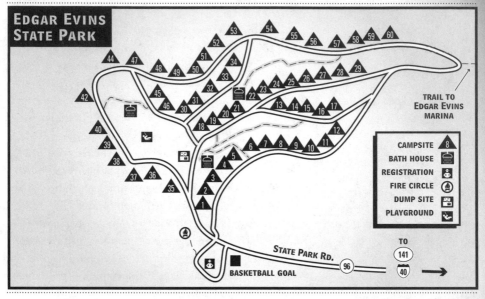

**EDGAR EVINS STATE PARK**

TRAIL TO
EDGAR EVINS
MARINA

| | |
|---|---|
| CAMPSITE | 8 |
| BATH HOUSE | |
| REGISTRATION | |
| FIRE CIRCLE | |
| DUMP SITE | |
| PLAYGROUND | |

TO
141
40

STATE PARK RD.

96

BASKETBALL GOAL

## GETTING THERE

From Exit 268 on I-40,
take TN 96 south
3.7 miles to the park.

# FALL CREEK FALLS STATE PARK

> *Fall Creek Falls is widely considered to be Tennessee's premier state park. The walk-in tent sites here certainly are the best anywhere.*

**T IS ONLY FITTING THAT FALL CREEK FALLS,** considered by many to be not only Tennessee's best state park, but one of the finest in the Southeast, would of course have some of the best walk-in tent campsites around. This 20,000-acre preserve is, however, more widely known for its natural features, such as its verdant old-growth forests punctuated with rock outcrops and sandstone bluffs overlooking steep gorges, and of course clear streams that fall to circular pools, giving this park atop the Cumberland Plateau its name. There are activities galore inside the park—if you can't do it here, you probably can't do it anywhere.

What about these great walk-in tent sites? They are a fairly recent addition to the park. It's a great thing for tent campers, because the main campground doesn't even begin to meet the high standards of beauty set here. The campground ratings in this book describe the walk-in sites only. If the rest of the campground were included, the ratings would be much lower. Suffice it to say that a maze of overcrowded sites is situated among too many loops. Sure, some decent sites are tucked away in the mix, but with these walk-in tent sites available I wouldn't bother. On the plus side, some of the primary sites can be reserved, but that only testifies to how busy the main campground is. Sometimes it seems like you are in a small city-of-the-woods.

The path to the walk-in sites starts behind the E Loop bathhouse. The trail immediately splits. The right trail heads past the only close walk-in site before dipping down a hollow. It then reaches a flat in a pine-and-oak forest with a well-groomed site off to the right. Drop down toward another hollow and come to two more sites that are so widely separated you can't see one from the other. The farthest site is about 150 yards from the car. The left-hand trail leads to farther campsites. Drop down to a fern hollow then climb a hill.

## RATINGS

Beauty: ☆ ☆ ☆ ☆ ☆
Privacy: ☆ ☆ ☆ ☆ ☆
Spaciousness: ☆ ☆ ☆ ☆ ☆
Quiet: ☆ ☆ ☆ ☆
Security: ☆ ☆ ☆ ☆
Cleanliness: ☆ ☆ ☆

Here is the first of five sites that are so far apart you begin to wonder if they are really out here. They are, and they are good. Walk-in campers use the E Loop bathhouse. During my midweek midsummer stay, the campground was nearly full, while only one of the nine walk-in sites was occupied. The walk-in sites cannot be reserved. On weekends, water- and electricity-loving campers will take walk-in sites out of desperation. Barring summer holidays, you can get a walk-in site during the week and on Fridays on summer weekends. During shoulder seasons getting a site is easy. I recommend coming to see the fall colors.

What should you do first? Start by heading to the Nature Center, which has displays about the park inside. Then get a trail map and visit the falls. Cross Cane Fork on a swinging bridge above a cascade. The pool below this cascade serves as a summertime swimming hole (the park does have a regulation swimming pool). Take the Gorge Trail to observe Cane Creek Falls, then check out gorge overlooks before coming to Fall Creek Falls. You can curve around and walk to the base of this 256-foot drop. Longer trails include the nearby Paw-Paw Trail and two long loops for overnight backpackers. Fall Creek Lake makes a pretty impoundment in the upper Fall Creek valley. Rent canoes, pedal boats, or johnboats. No gas motors are allowed, but fishing is, and it is reputed to be good.

If you don't feel like walking, ride a bike. Bikes are for rent at Village Green Area, where a recreation hall, visitors lounge, and park information center stand. Take a trail ride at the park stables or make a scenic drive. The one-way Gorge Scenic Drive circles the Cane Creek Gorge then heads up Piney Creek Gorge where you can check out Piney Creek Falls. Park naturalists conduct nature programs. Kids 12 and under have their own programs. Take a pontoon boat ride, tour Camp's Branch Cave, or go on a group bike ride. There are ball courts for conventional games such as tennis, softball, and basketball. If you don't feel like cooking, grab a meal at the park restaurant where they have breakfast, lunch, and dinner buffets. Come to think of it, a trip to Fall Creek Falls could be called an outdoor buffet.

## KEY INFORMATION

**ADDRESS:** Route 3, Box 300 Pikeville, TN 37367

**OPERATED BY:** Tennessee State Parks

**INFORMATION:** (423) 881-3297; reservations (800) 250-8611

**OPEN:** Year-round

**SITES:** 9 walk-in tent sites, 228 others

**EACH SITE HAS:** Picnic table, fire ring, lantern post, tent pad (walk-in sites); water and electricity (other sites)

**ASSIGNMENT:** Walk-in sites are first come, first served and do not take reservations; some others can be reserved

**REGISTRATION:** At camper registration station

**FACILITIES:** Hot showers, flush toilets, water spigots, laundry, pay phone, camp store

**PARKING:** At walk-in parking area and at campsites

**FEE:** $8 per night walk-in tent sites; $17 per night other

**ELEVATION:** 1,700 feet

**RESTRICTIONS:** Pets: On 6-foot leash only
Fires: In fire rings only
Alcohol: Prohibited
Vehicles: None
Other: Maximum 14-day stay

# MAP

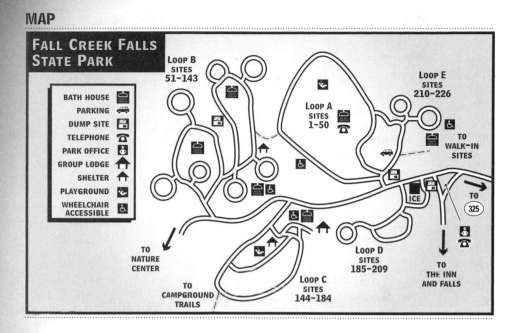

**FALL CREEK FALLS STATE PARK**

LOOP B
SITES
51-143

LOOP A
SITES
1-50

LOOP E
SITES
210-226

TO
WALK-IN
SITES

BATH HOUSE
PARKING
DUMP SITE
TELEPHONE
PARK OFFICE
GROUP LODGE
SHELTER
PLAYGROUND
WHEELCHAIR
ACCESSIBLE

ICE

TO
325

TO
NATURE
CENTER

LOOP D
SITES
185-209

TO
THE INN
AND FALLS

TO
CAMPGROUND
TRAILS

LOOP C
SITES
144-184

## GETTING THERE

From Pikeville, head 12 miles west on TN 30 to TN 284. Turn left on TN 284 and travel a little over 4 miles to reach the campers' registration booth. The walk-in tent sites are nearby.

# GATLIN POINT

**T**HIS IS A BOATER'S CAMPGROUND, which is only fitting for a camp located at Land Between The Lakes (LBL) National Recreation Area. Gatlin Point Campground overlooks two lakes—Bards Lake and Lake Barkley. However, only a low dam over which a paved road is laid separates these lakes. A north-facing wooded hill overlooking both impoundments is the setting for this campground. Continue straight on the access road and turn left into the campground just before reaching the dam. Three campsites are located near the lake and are shaded by the afternoon sun. These are the most popular sites. Another two sites are located in the open, in a grassy area overlooking the lake. They offer good views but no privacy. There are additional tiered sites up the hill; these are shaded by oaks of varying ages and a few cedars. A grassy understory complements the sites, which are a little close together. But since this is an underutilized campground, you likely won't have to worry about there being neighbors nearby. There are additional secluded sites away from the lake. Of special note is campsite 19, tucked away along an intermittent stream. The campground has two reliable water spigots as well as portable toilets.

Bards Lake, at 320 acres, is divided from Lake Barkley by the dam visible from the campground. This is a no-wake lake with a primitive gravel launch at the low point of the campground. Canoers and kayakers will especially enjoy smaller Bards Lake, which is less windy than Lake Barkley and has no current to battle. Gatlin Point is the terminus for the Land Between The Lakes Paddle Route, which starts at Boswell Landing on Kentucky Lake to the west and circles the entire

> *Enjoy two bodies of water from one campground!*

## RATINGS

Beauty: ✩ ✩ ✩
Privacy: ✩ ✩ ✩
Spaciousness: ✩ ✩ ✩ ✩
Quiet: ✩ ✩ ✩ ✩
Security: ✩ ✩
Cleanliness: ✩ ✩ ✩

**ADDRESS:** 100 Van Morgan
Drive
Golden Pond, KY
42211

**OPERATED BY:** Land Between The
Lakes National
Recreation Area

**INFORMATION:** (800) LBL-7077;
www.lbl.org

**OPEN:** Year-round

**SITES:** 24

**EACH SITE HAS:** Picnic table, fire
grate

**ASSIGNMENT:** First come, first
served; no
reservations

**REGISTRATION:** Self-registration
on-site

**FACILITIES:** Water spigot,
portable toilet

**PARKING:** At campsites only

**FEE:** $8 per night,
decreasing with
each consecutive
night of stay

**ELEVATION:** 520 feet

**RESTRICTIONS:** Pets: On leash only
Fires: In fire rings
only
Alcohol: At
campsites only
Vehicles: None
Other: Maximum
14-day stay

Land Between The Lakes Peninsula to end here at Gatlin Point, a trip of nearly 100 miles that tempts intrepid kayakers. Anglers in smaller boats will enjoy the scenery of Bards Lake and may find a few fish on the end of their lines. The grassy setting of Brandon Spring Group Center is visible across Bards Lake. A bona fide, concrete boat-launch is located on the far side of the dam, allowing motorboat access to Lake Barkley. At this point, Lake Barkley resembles a long strand of water broken by several small ribbonlike islands. If you want to stretch your legs, gated fire roads spur from the campground and can serve as informal trails.

Despite being a boater's campground, Gatlin Point has good hiking nearby, including Bear Creek Loop. This 6.6-mile circuit, one of the best at LBL, leaves the picnic area across from the intersection of the Trace and Fort Henry Road just north of the South Welcome Station that you passed on the way in. Head south on Telegraph Trail and dip into the Bear Creek watershed to see some of the best wildflower displays at LBL. Pass old homesites and fields along Dry Branch before climbing onto a ridgeline. Turn north on the Fort Henry North–South Trail Connector past meadows to meet the North–South Trail. Return to the picnic area after traversing an attractive woodland. Another good loop, the 7.4-mile Model Loop Trail, lies to the north. This trek passes old homesites, springs, and a bison range. It starts near the Homeplace, a good destination for history buffs who want to learn about the pioneer life in this part of Tennessee. Supplies can be had in nearby Dover. I highly recommend visiting Fort Donelson National Battlefield when you pass this way. It offers insight into the Civil War in Tennessee, good hiking, and great views of Lake Barkley, which will make you understand why this locale was chosen as a fort. The battlefield is located just west of Dover.

# MAP

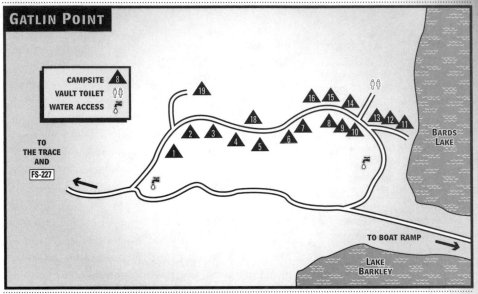

GATLIN POINT

CAMPSITE ▲8
VAULT TOILET
WATER ACCESS

TO THE TRACE AND FS-227

BARDS LAKE

TO BOAT RAMP

LAKE BARKLEY

## GETTING THERE

From Dover, take US 79
south to the Trace. Turn right
on the Trace to reach
the South Welcome Station
after 3.4 miles. Continue
north on the Trace 0.9 miles
farther to FR 227. Turn right
on FR 227 and follow it
2 miles. Veer left on FR 229
and follow it 1.5 miles.
The campground will be
on your left.

# HARPETH RIVER BRIDGE

> *This is a great tent campground for enjoying both Cheatham Lake and the lower Harpeth River.*

**H**ARPETH RIVER BRIDGE CAMPGROUND is strategically located at the mouth of the Harpeth River where it flows into the now-dammed Cumberland River, known as Cheatham Lake at this juncture. This makes for watery recreation opportunities in both the flowing Harpeth, a state scenic river, and the narrow Cheatham Lake. Because the campground was constructed by the Army Corps of Engineers, it is well built and in great shape. The nearby and more popular Lock 1 Campground, also an Army Corps of Engineers venue, overlooks Harpeth Bridge. Leave TN 49 and descend to a flat beside the Harpeth River. Pass the entrance station and campground-host campsite to enter a loop. Campsites 2 through 5 are located fairly near one another and back up to a cove of Cheatham Lake, still water that would be good for canoeing. Curve around the loop to reach campsite 6, which is by a little creek connecting to the Harpeth River. The riverside campsites start with 8. The first few campsites are a little too open to the sun. But there are plenty of shady riverside sites as you head past campsites up to campsite 14. A boat ramp leading into the Harpeth River extends to the water beyond campsite 14. Bathrooms are located on the last part of the loop.

Riverine Cheatham Lake covers 7,450 acres and has 320 miles of shoreline. Many interesting fingers and arms, including the embayment of the Harpeth River, provide good wildlife habitat. A small johnboat is good for exploring these often-shallow waters where anglers fish for largemouth bass. Anglers on the shore or the campground's bank can catch bream and crappie with worms and other bait. Other people use bait to catch catfish. Canoeing the Harpeth River has always been a favorite Middle Tennessee pastime of mine. You can make a trip of 12 miles by starting

## RATINGS

Beauty: ☆ ☆ ☆
Privacy: ☆ ☆ ☆
Spaciousness: ☆ ☆ ☆ ☆
Quiet: ☆ ☆
Security: ☆ ☆ ☆ ☆ ☆
Cleanliness: ☆ ☆ ☆ ☆

at the TN 250 bridge and floating down to the campground.

Farther upstream and accessible by car is Narrows of Harpeth State Historic Area. You can hike and canoe here where the Harpeth River, in a 5-mile-long bend, nearly curves back on itself. One trail heads upstream along the Harpeth then descends to a man-made tunnel that cuts across the bend in the river. Montgomery Bell built the tunnel to harness the water-power of the Harpeth for his iron forge. Back in the early 1800s Bell was developing the iron-ore industry in Middle Tennessee and was looking for a place to build a water-powered mill on the Harpeth River; he noticed where the Harpeth made such a bend that it nearly doubled back on itself, separated only by slender but steep bluff. What took a person in a boat 5 miles by water took a person on foot a half hour to clamber over. In those 5 miles, the Harpeth dropped several feet. Bell saw the chance to use water power, diverted from the river and through a tunnel, for his iron-ore industry if he could cut through that bluff. Using slave labor Bell started the project in 1819, boring the tunnel through the limestone bluff that is 8 feet high, 16 feet wide, and 290 feet long. The ironworks around the Narrows are long gone, but water still flows through the tunnel. Today you can float this 5-mile segment of the Harpeth without a shuttle: the beginning and ending points of the float are just a short walk apart. You can also hike to a high bluff atop the Narrows for a panoramic view of the Harpeth River and surrounding countryside.

To access the Narrows of Harpeth from Harpeth River Bridge Campground, take TN 49 back toward Ashland City, then turn right on TN 249 and follow it to US 70. Turn right onto US 70 and follow it to Cedar Hill Road. Turn right on Cedar Hill Road and follow it 3 miles to the Harris Street Bridge, which will be on your right. Turn right into a parking area just before the bridge. A trail starts down by the Harpeth River beyond some vehicle-barrier boulders. After your hike you can return to Harpeth River Bridge Campground.

## MAP

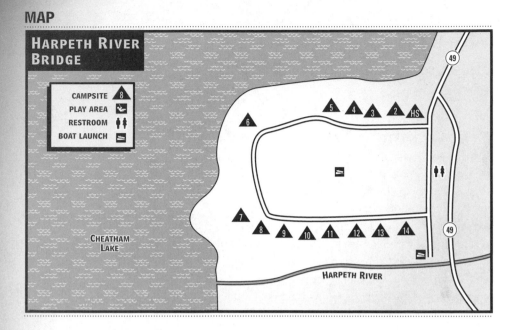

# HARPETH RIVER BRIDGE

| | |
|---|---|
| CAMPSITE | 8 |
| PLAY AREA | |
| RESTROOM | |
| BOAT LAUNCH | |

49

5 4 3 2 HS

6

CHEATHAM LAKE

7

8 9 10 11 12 13 14

49

HARPETH RIVER

## GETTING THERE

From Ashland City, take TN 49 south to the campground, which is on your right just before the bridge over the Harpeth River.

# HENRY HORTON STATE PARK

**H**ENRY **HORTON IS CLASSIFIED** as a state resort park, which means it has a golf course, a lodge, cabins, and more. However, for tent campers and outdoor-recreation enthusiasts, Henry Horton has another side—the side that has two tent-camping areas and the beauty of the Duck River, with its massive rock bluffs and tree-lined banks. The Duck, an appealing canoeing stream, flows through the heart of the park, dividing the resort side of the park from the more rustic part that appeals to tent campers. So pitch your tent and then head down the Duck for a fun Middle Tennessee float trip.

The fairly large campground here has two areas for tent campers—the tent area and the wilderness area. Using the word "wilderness" is stretching it a bit, but this nine-site area is ideal for tent campers. It is set apart from the rest of the campground on its own gravel side road, which separates a field from dense woods. The ground is level here beneath the forest of oak, hickory, and cedar. Smaller trees such as dogwood form a dense understory, and many rock outcrops add scenic beauty to the campsites. The campsites are large and spaced well apart from one another as they stretch out along the gravel road. There is a small auto turnaround at the end of the road. A second area for tent campers lies near the Duck River at the beginning of the main campground. These nine sites are laid out on another gravel road with a small spur near one of the bathhouses. The whole area dips toward the Duck River. The campsites are shady here but don't have the dense understory that the Wilderness Camp has. This understory is grassier.

The main campground is laid out in a large paved loop in a shady woodland. There are both pull-in and

> *The Wilderness Camp adds to the appeal of this park on the banks of the Duck River.*

## RATINGS

Beauty: ☆ ☆ ☆
Privacy: ☆ ☆ ☆ ☆ ☆
Spaciousness: ☆ ☆ ☆ ☆
Quiet: ☆ ☆ ☆
Security: ☆ ☆ ☆ ☆ ☆
Cleanliness: ☆ ☆ ☆ ☆

**ADDRESS:** P.O. Box 128 Chapel Hill, TN 37034

**OPERATED BY:** Tennessee State Parks

**INFORMATION:** (931) 364-2222; www.tnstateparks.com

**OPEN:** Year-round

**SITES:** 9 tent sites, 9 wilderness tent sites, 54 RV sites

**EACH SITE HAS:** picnic table, fire grate (Wilderness Camp and Tent Camp); picnic table, upright grill, fire grate, water, electricity (rest of campground)

**ASSIGNMENT:** First come, first served; no reservations

**REGISTRATION:** Campground host will register you

**FACILITIES:** Hot showers, flush toilets, pay phone

**PARKING:** At campsites only

**FEE:** $10.75 per night tent sites, $6.75 per night wilderness sites, $17 per night RV sites

**ELEVATION:** 600 feet

**RESTRICTIONS:** Pets: On 6-foot leash only
Fires: In fire rings only
Alcohol: Prohibited
Vehicles: Maximum 2 vehicles per site
Other: Maximum 14-day stay

pull-through sites on the slightly hilly terrain. The sites are more pinched in toward the end of the loop. For the most part, this area is for RVs; leave it for them. I recommend the wilderness sites over all the rest. They are near-ideal sites for tent campers and are also the cheapest. The park, which has a campground host, fills on summer holiday weekends and during occasional nearby special events.

Named after the 36th governor of Tennessee, the land for this park was donated by the Wilhoite family, into which ol' Henry Horton married. It offers a little bit of everything for visitors. Here is a quick rundown of activities: tennis, badminton, basketball, disc golf, volleyball, and skeet shooting. The camp also has an Olympic-sized pool with lifeguards on duty in summer. On the more rustic side is Turkey Trail, which makes a 2.5-mile loop for hikers to enjoy. The Wilhoite Mill Trail, where Henry's relatives ground their meal, courses along the Duck River past machine relics from days gone by. Small side trails lead to bluffs overlooking the Duck River and to swimming and fishing access points. Hickory Ridge Nature Loop, a shorter trail, starts near the wilderness camping area and connects to the park nature center, where a park recreation director, on duty in summer, has all sorts of activities for kids and adults alike, from horseback riding to hay rides. Call ahead for a list of weekly activities.

Many folks come to Henry Horton not only to camp but also to float the Duck River. A nearby outfitter makes this pastime convenient for those who don't have their own canoe or are looking to be shuttled from the takeout back to their car upriver. Duck River Canoe Rental at Forest Landing is just north of the park on US 31A. It offers a fine day trip from Hopkins Bridge to the state park. Choose a canoe or kayak and float fishfor bass or bream, take a dip in the water, or just enjoy the riverside sights. For reservations, call (931) 364-7874. Also reserve some time for a tent-camping excursion to Henry Horton State Park.

# MAP

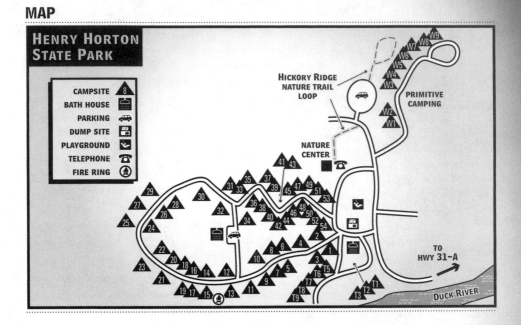

**HENRY HORTON STATE PARK**

| | |
|---|---|
| CAMPSITE | 8 |
| BATH HOUSE | |
| PARKING | |
| DUMP SITE | |
| PLAYGROUND | |
| TELEPHONE | |
| FIRE RING | |

HICKORY RIDGE
NATURE TRAIL
LOOP

NATURE
CENTER

PRIMITIVE
CAMPING

W9
W8
W7
W6
W5
W4
W3
W2
W1

TO
HWY 31-A

DUCK RIVER

## GETTING THERE

From Exit 46 on I-65 near Columbia, head 13 miles east on TN 99 to US 31A. Turn right onto 31A and follow it 2 miles south to the state park, which will be on your right.

# LILLYDALE

> *The island walk-in tent sites are the best among many good campsites at this campground on Dale Hollow Lake.*

**MANY PEOPLE ARGUE THAT** Dale Hollow Lake is the prettiest lake in Tennessee, if not in the entire South. Backed against the western edge of the Cumberland Plateau, the impoundment is bordered by hills, coves, islands, and fingers, a combination of land and water that is very easy on the eyes. The lower Obey River Valley was flooded to create this lake on Tennessee's northern border, so far north that it extends into Kentucky, with the Bluegrass State claiming part of it as its own. And who can blame them? Fortunately for us, when the Army Corps of Engineers created Dale Hollow Lake, they also created many recreation areas, and Lillydale is among the best, especially for us Tennessee tent campers.

What makes Lillydale so good? For starters it is a well-built and well-maintained facility. The campsites are very large and well separated from one another. They are in good shape, and campground hosts are on site full-time to make sure things run smoothly. But I think the best reason to stay here are the walk-in tent campsites located on an island in Dale Hollow Lake! More about them later.

The rest of the campground is located on a hilly peninsula that juts into Dale Hollow Lake. Descend past the tollhouse, and the expanse of the campground opens before you. Lake vistas are everywhere! The first camping area, with sites 1 through 16, is on the right. These campsites are of special note because they are the best ones for tent campers. Shade is minimal here because the trees are young. At some sites you park your car then walk down steps to lakefront camps that overlook the water below. Reservations should be made for sites 8 through 15. Bring a sun shelter because shade is lacking. The next area, 16 through 46, is good for tent campers who want to be near their cars. It is higher on the peninsula and has many

## RATINGS

Beauty: ☆ ☆ ☆ ☆
Privacy: ☆ ☆ ☆
Spaciousness: ☆ ☆ ☆ ☆ ☆
Quiet: ☆ ☆ ☆
Security: ☆ ☆ ☆ ☆ ☆
Cleanliness: ☆ ☆ ☆ ☆

lakefront sites with million-dollar views. As is normally the case, the lakefront sites go first.

A land bridge connects the main campground to the camping island. The island, with sites 101 through 115, is mostly grassy with scattered trees. All the campsites are on the edge of the island. Young trees provide a little shade—bring a sun shelter. The island is large and is a good hoof from the walk-in tent parking area. Many campers load their boats then boat around to their campsites on the edge of the island. The views from the large and spacious sites are great. I highly recommend these campsites; they are among the best in this entire guidebook.

The campground, back on the mainland, is arranged in concentric loops; all have electricity. Most of these sites are not for tent campers, but those who want lakefront sites with electricity can find them here. Two modern bathhouses serve the campground.

Lillydale Campground has its own recreational facilities. A basketball court and a volleyball court are adjacent to the island camp, as is a swim beach. And the campground has its own boat ramp. However, with so many lakefront campsites, many visitors keep their boats tied up directly in front of their camp. Additionally, the 8-mile Accordion Bluff Trail connects Lillydale Recreation Area with the nearby Willow Grove Recreation Area.

Most campers come here to enjoy water recreation on this pretty lake. Fishing, boating, skiing, and swimming are the most popular pastimes. Lillydale is primarily a warm-weather experience, and the area can be busy on summer weekends, so you might as well join in the fun rather than seek peace and quiet here: you won't find any. So load up your water toys and head up to Lillydale. A word of advice: There is only a small convenience store nearby, so get the bulk of your supplies before you come here, as it is a fair piece back to civilization on slow two-lane roads.

## KEY INFORMATION

**ADDRESS:** 5050 Dale Hollow Dam Road Celina, TN 38551

**OPERATED BY:** Army Corps of Engineers

**INFORMATION:** (931) 243-3136 or www.lrn.usace.army.mil; reservation information (877) 444-6777 or www.reserveusa.com

**OPEN:** May–Labor Day weekend

**SITES:** 15 walk-in island tent campsites, 99 other sites

**EACH SITE HAS:** Picnic table, fire ring, upright grill, lantern post, tent pad; some also have electricity

**ASSIGNMENT:** First come, first served; reservations available

**REGISTRATION:** At campground entrance station

**FACILITIES:** Hot showers, flush toilets, laundry, telephone

**PARKING:** At campsites and at walk-in tent camping area

**FEE:** $8 to $22 per night depending on proximity to water and electricity

**ELEVATION:** 850 feet

**RESTRICTIONS:** Pets: On 6-foot leash only
Fires: In fire rings only
Alcohol: At campsites only
Vehicles: None
Other: Maximum 14-day stay in a 30-day period

## MAP

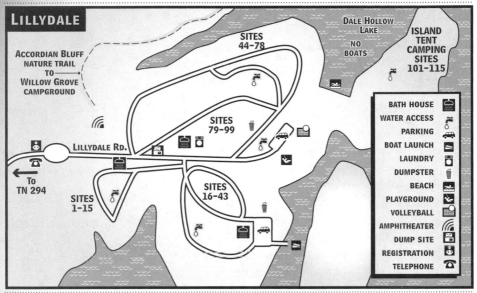

**LILLYDALE**

ACCORDIAN BLUFF
NATURE TRAIL
TO
WILLOW GROVE
CAMPGROUND

SITES
44-78

DALE HOLLOW
LAKE

NO
BOATS

ISLAND
TENT
CAMPING
SITES
101-115

SITES
79-99

LILLYDALE RD.

To
TN 294

SITES
1-15

SITES
16-43

BATH HOUSE
WATER ACCESS
PARKING
BOAT LAUNCH
LAUNDRY
DUMPSTER
BEACH
PLAYGROUND
VOLLEYBALL
AMPHITHEATER
DUMP SITE
REGISTRATION
TELEPHONE

## GETTING THERE

From Livingston, stay on TN
111 north to TN 294 north.
Turn left onto TN 294 north
and follow it 13.7 miles to
Lillydale Road. Turn right
onto Lillydale Road and follow it 1 mile to the dead end
at the recreation area.

# MERIWETHER LEWIS MONUMENT

**T**HIS IS ONE CAMPGROUND WHERE you will want to take your time heading to it, traveling the Natchez Trace Parkway, of course. I came from Nashville and stopped at the many roadside sights. Upon arriving at Meriwether Lewis Monument Campground, set on a wooded ridge, I found an added bonus: free camping! My overall experience was so good that I was almost ashamed I hadn't experienced it before. In addition to the interesting human and natural history, as well as free camping, the nearby Buffalo River offers one of the finest canoe float trips in the state.

The campground sits on a ridgetop in young oak and hickory woods. It is comprised of one loop and a side road. Steep hillsides drop off from all sides. Younger trees, some of which are dogwoods, separate the sites. The camping areas are well maintained and well spaced and offer decent privacy. The other camping area is on a narrow side ridge, with sites strung along the road. Each site has a good view into the woods below. This area has the only bathrooms in the campground. But who's complaining? The campground is free! A small auto turnaround at the end of the road offers a few more sites that are the quietest of all.

There is a water spigot at each camping area, and a campground host. Campers can get a site almost any time of year. A few weeks in March, April, October, and November are the only times the campground is full: this is when snowbirds from up north are heading to or from their winter destinations. Otherwise, Meriwether Lewis is the domain of tenters.

The Natchez Trace came to be when boatmen returning from delivering crops and other goods down the Cumberland, Ohio, and Mississippi rivers began returning to their homes via a buffalo and native Indian path running from Natchez, Mississippi, to

> *The Natchez Trace Parkway is lined with interesting historical sights and features a free campground.*

## RATINGS

Beauty: ✪ ✪ ✪ ✪
Privacy: ✪ ✪ ✪ ✪
Spaciousness: ✪ ✪ ✪
Quiet: ✪ ✪ ✪ ✪
Security: ✪ ✪ ✪ ✪ ✪
Cleanliness: ✪ ✪ ✪ ✪ ✪

| | |
|---|---|
| **ADDRESS:** | 2680 Natchez Trace Parkway Tupelo, MS 38801 |
| **OPERATED BY:** | National Park Service |
| **INFORMATION:** | (800) 305-7417; www.nps.gov/natr |
| **OPEN:** | Year-round |
| **SITES:** | 32 |
| **EACH SITE HAS:** | Picnic table, fire ring |
| **ASSIGNMENT:** | First come, first served; no reservations |
| **REGISTRATION:** | No registration |
| **FACILITIES:** | Water spigot, flush toilets |
| **PARKING:** | At campsites only |
| **FEE:** | No fee |
| **ELEVATION:** | 900 feet |
| **RESTRICTIONS:** | Pets: On 6-foot leash only Fires: In fire rings only Alcohol: At campsites only Vehicles: None Other: Maximum 14-day stay |

Nashville, Tennessee. The federal government then commissioned roadwork, improving the path. The Natchez Trace became one of our first western roads. Portions of this old road are actually preserved to this day and can be walked on. You'll have to learn the rest of the story on your own. One of my favorite sights along the parkway is the Gordon House, built in 1812. Mr. Gordon operated a ferry on the Duck River. Down the road is the preserved relic of an old tobacco farm, with great views from the ridgeline. Jackson Falls, a two-tiered fall that drops over a rock rim, exhibits some of the natural beauty of the region. A trail leads down the falls and another cascade coming from a side creek. There are many more places to visit north and south of Meriwether Lewis Monument.

Here, near the campground, is the actual monument to Meriwether Lewis (as in Lewis and Clark), one of the leaders of the famous Corps of Discovery expedition that went up the Missouri River and overland to the Pacific in the early 1800s. After the expedition, Lewis died here under circumstances that remain one of the great mysteries in American history. He is buried at the monument.

Several miles of trails run along the ridges and hollows in the immediate area. Get a trail map at the log cabin near the monument. There is a longer hike north of here on the Natchez Trace National Scenic Trail. It runs 26 miles near Gordon House, north of the campground. Check out the picnic area at Little Swan Creek, an attractive stream with small bluffs along its clear waters. A bigger waterway is the Buffalo River, which flows free 110 miles past large bluffs that look out over good fishing waters. Some of my most memorable paddling trips have been here. Fish for smallmouth bass or bream. Or just enjoy the scenery. Call (800) 339-5596 for an outfitter in nearby Hohenwald.

# MAP

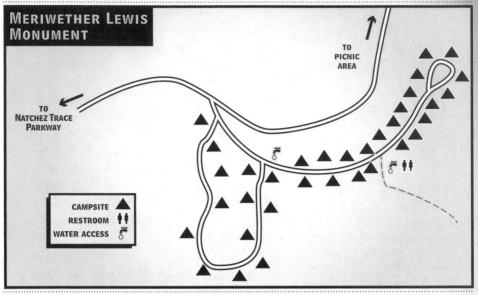

**MERIWETHER LEWIS MONUMENT**

TO
PICNIC
AREA

TO
NATCHEZ TRACE
PARKWAY

CAMPSITE
RESTROOM
WATER ACCESS

## GETTING THERE

From Columbia, take TN 50
west 15 miles to the
Natchez Trace Parkway.
Head south on the parkway
22 miles to Meriwether
Lewis Monument, which will
be on your right.

# MONTGOMERY BELL STATE PARK

> *This popular campground is convenient to Nashville.*

**M**ONTGOMERY BELL WAS A Middle Tennessee mover and shaker back in the early 1800s. He moved to Dickson County to work in the burgeoning iron-ore industry and actually extracted the ore that would be used in cannonballs at the Battle of New Orleans in 1812. Bell recognized the natural beauty of the area, beyond its economic appeal, as did later Tennesseans who established this state park. Today you can enjoy the popular campground, hiking trails, and other features and facilities that comprise this state park.

The campground is large but well laid out in a flat along the banks of Hall Creek. Pass the camper check-in station and turn right onto the main loop. This begins the area of tent sites, where a tall cedar and hardwood forest provides shade. The tent sites in the center of the loop are in a parklike setting. This area is very level, and the sites are spacious, but a merely grassy understory minimizes campsite privacy. Some sites on the outside of the loop are a little too sloped for a good night's sleep. A crossroad with more tent sites bisects the main loop, which swings around toward Hall Creek. All the sites are alluring, save for a few more hillside ones. Then the main loop comes along Hall Creek and the end of the tent sites. However, the campsites along Hall Creek are also open to tent campers. These sites are fairly large and offer access to the clear stream that overlies flat slabs of limestone. There is a bluff across the creek from the campsites.

Sites continue along both sides of the main campground loop. The farther upstream, the more RVs. Beyond the main loop is one more loop that is wide open to the sun, with campsites that are too close together. Avoid these. Three bathhouses are spread along the campground. Tent campers will seek out sites 51 through 104.

## RATINGS

Beauty: ✩ ✩ ✩
Privacy: ✩ ✩ ✩
Spaciousness: ✩ ✩ ✩ ✩
Quiet: ✩ ✩ ✩ ✩
Security: ✩ ✩ ✩ ✩ ✩
Cleanliness: ✩ ✩ ✩ ✩ ✩

Montgomery Bell's proximity to Nashville makes it a convenient getaway for city residents but also sees the campground fill during the summer holidays and on warm-weather weekends. Try to get here early on Friday if you can. Better yet, come during the week. Our visit was on a warm summer weekday, and the campground had a sleepy feel to it. Hall Creek was lazily flowing to meet Jones Creek. We could have taken a nap but instead made a hiking loop out of the campground using a combination of trails. Even though it was mid-afternoon we came upon a deer and fawn, which were out and about despite the heat. The deer surprised us as we dipped into a hollow to continue to enjoy the shady woods. Later we had a picnic in lower Wildcat Hollow, looking at the park map and discussing what else we could do here. And there is plenty.

Lake Acorn has a swimming beach for cooling off after a hike like ours. If you love to be near the water but not in it, try a canoe, rowboat, or paddleboat. Many folks come here for catfish, bream, and bass. If Lake Acorn isn't producing, try the other park lakes: Woodhaven and Creech Hollow.

Game players can try croquet, shuffleboard, volleyball, and tennis. Nature enthusiasts can enjoy the park's trail system. The master trail is the Montgomery Bell Trail, which makes an 11.5-mile loop through the park. A cross trail, Creech Hollow, makes 5-mile loop hikes possible on the Montgomery Bell Trail. Shorter paths include the Ore Pit Trail, which examines the mining history of the park, and the J. Bailey Trail, which makes a loop near the park's headquarters. Campers use the Wildcat Trail to leave the campground to connect to the Montgomery Bell Trail and others. In summer, park naturalists are on hand, offering campfire programs and nature presentations as well as more kid-oriented activities such as arts and crafts. I can't say for sure, but I believe Montgomery Bell would be proud of this state park named in his honor.

## KEY INFORMATION

| | |
|---|---|
| **ADDRESS:** | P.O. Box 39 Burns, TN 37029 |
| **OPERATED BY:** | Tennessee State Parks |
| **INFORMATION:** | (615) 797-9052; www.tnstateparks.com |
| **OPEN:** | Year-round |
| **SITES:** | 27 tent; 94 water and electric |
| **EACH SITE HAS:** | Picnic table, fire ring |
| **ASSIGNMENT:** | First come, first served; no reservations |
| **REGISTRATION:** | At campground registration hut |
| **FACILITIES:** | Hot showers, flush toilets |
| **PARKING:** | At campsites only |
| **FEE:** | $11 per night tent sites, $17 per night water and electric sites |
| **ELEVATION:** | 650 feet |
| **RESTRICTIONS:** | Pets: On 6-foot leash only Fires: In fire rings only Alcohol: Prohibited Vehicles: Maximum 2 vehicles per site Other: Maximum 14-day stay |

# MAP

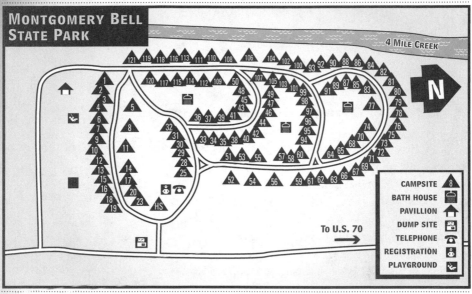

## GETTING THERE

From Exit 182 on I-40, head west 11 miles on TN 96 to US 70. Turn right onto US 70, then head 4 miles east to the state park entrance, which will be on the right.

# MOUSETAIL LANDING STATE PARK

*Parsons*

**M**OUSETAIL **LANDING.** What a name! No telling what you imagine earned it this name. Here's the story: Back in the 1800s, there was a tannery here on the Tennessee River. Being a tannery, it had many fresh animal hides on hand, which attracted mice. One day, a fire broke out at the tannery, and suddenly thousands of mice tore out of there. And that's how the river landing came to be known as Mousetail Landing. But don't worry, the mice are gone. Now there is instead a great state park with two good but different campgrounds for us to pitch our tents and enjoy the park's finer things, like swimming, fishing, boating, and backwoods hiking.

The Primitive Campground is the tenter's best choice. It is located on the Spring Creek embayment of the Tennessee River. A forest of shagbark hickory, sweetgum, winged elm, and various oaks shades the camping area. The first two campsites are on their own, then the campground road passes over a wet-weather drainage to enter a super-shady flat with large campsites before the road turns right. Several waterside camps with a grassy understory spur off the main road. Farther along, the sites become more spacious and heavily shaded and the main channel of the Tennessee River comes into view. A few open sites stand near the river. Directly beside the Tennessee is a picnic area and grassy lawn with a few trees interspersed. Here campers can watch the tugboats pass as they push barges up and down the mighty waterway. Campers who stay here can use the bathhouse at the Main Campground.

The Main Campground is in the park proper, a mile or so from the Primitive Campground. It is located high on a wooded ridge. Its 25 sites are spread out along three mini-loops. The first loop is for tenters and has no water or electricity. A mixture of grass and

> *Both waterside and hilltop sites await you by the Tennessee River.*

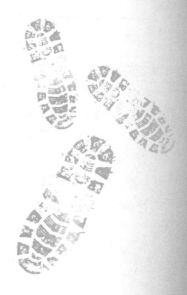

## RATINGS

Beauty: ✿ ✿ ✿ ✿
Privacy: ✿ ✿ ✿
Spaciousness: ✿ ✿ ✿ ✿
Quiet: ✿ ✿ ✿ ✿
Security: ✿ ✿ ✿ ✿
Cleanliness: ✿ ✿ ✿ ✿ ✿

## KEY INFORMATION

**ADDRESS:** Route 3, Box 280B
Linden, TN 37096

**OPERATED BY:** Tennessee State
Parks

**INFORMATION:** (731) 847-0841;
www.tnstateparks.
com

**OPEN:** Year-round

**SITES:** 46

**EACH SITE HAS:** Picnic table, lantern
post, upright grill,
fire ring (Primitive
Area); water,
electricity, picnic
table, upright grill
(Main Area)

**ASSIGNMENT:** First come, first
served; no
reservations

**REGISTRATION:** Ranger will come
by to register you

**FACILITIES:** Hot showers and
water spigots at
Main Area; vault
toilets at Primitive
Area

**PARKING:** At campsites only

**FEE:** Primitive Camp-
ground $12 per
night; Main Camp-
ground $12 per
night nonelectric
sites, $16 per night
electric sites

**ELEVATION:** Primitive Campground 360 feet;
Main Campground
580 feet

**RESTRICTIONS:** Pets: On 6-foot
leash only
Fires: In fire rings
only
Alcohol: Prohib-
ited
Vehicles: Maxi-
mum 2 tents per
site
Other: Maximum
14-day stay

trees make it more open. The hillside drops off steeply from the edge of the campsites that have been leveled with landscaping timbers. Tent pads have been installed, too. Pass the modern bathhouse to come to the next loop, where the sites have water and electricity. Hickories shade this camping area. The third loop has ten sites and is more shaded still. The small dead-end side road has a few desirable sites. Vegetation has been added wherever the sites lacked privacy.

I stayed in the Primitive Campground on my visit. Spring was breaking loose, and it seemed the trees were greening before my very eyes. Late in the evening I walked out to the water and watched the sun set as a barge chugged around the bend. Most folks bring their own boats during the warmer months, pulling them right up to the riverside sites. There is a swimming beach at the main park, and you are welcome to swim at your own risk. Fishing for catfish, bass, and bream is popular year-round.

Back on land, the Day Use Trail makes a 3-mile loop from the park office down toward the river and up Sparks Ridge. This trail can also be accessed by a spur trail from near the campground. Hardier hikers will want to tackle the Eagle Point Loop. It runs up Kelly Hollow, over Sparks Ridge, down to Parrish Branch, then to near the original Mousetail Landing. From there it ascends a bluff to afford hikers a great view. The trail then skirts along the Lick Creek embayment before climbing a steep hill to complete the 8-mile loop.

Just outside the park is another hike, this one offering a great view from Lady Finger Bluff in a Tennessee Valley Area Small Wild Area. A trail map and directions are available at the park office. Start on the far side of Lick Creek Embayment and make a 3-mile trek to a rock outcrop framed in gnarled, old red cedar trees. Here you'll have a sweeping view of the Tennessee River. Whether it is from Lady Finger Bluff or the Primitive Campground, the view will make you agree that this part of the Volunteer State is a good place to be.

## MAP

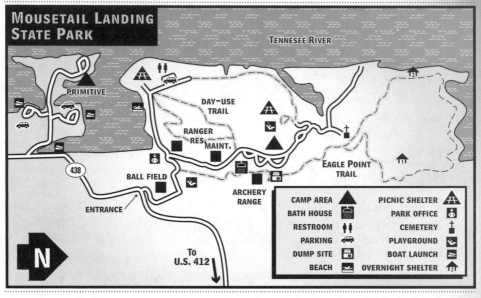

### MOUSETAIL LANDING STATE PARK

TENNESEE RIVER

PRIMITIVE

DAY-USE TRAIL

RANGER RES.
MAINT.

438

BALL FIELD

ENTRANCE

ARCHERY RANGE

EAGLE POINT TRAIL

To U.S. 412

N

| CAMP AREA | PICNIC SHELTER |
| BATH HOUSE | PARK OFFICE |
| RESTROOM | CEMETERY |
| PARKING | PLAYGROUND |
| DUMP SITE | BOAT LAUNCH |
| BEACH | OVERNIGHT SHELTER |

## GETTING THERE

From Parsons, drive 10 miles east on US 412 to TN 438. Turn left and follow TN 438 east 2.1 miles to the state park, on your left.

# OLD STONE FORT STATE ARCHEOLOGICAL PARK

> *The tableland between the Duck and Little Duck rivers has been regarded as special for thousands of years.*

**T**HIS STATE ARCHEOLOGICAL PARK preserves a 2,000-year-old native Indian ceremonial site on a 50-acre swath between the Little Duck and Duck rivers. We may never know what was the exact purpose of this area, which is enclosed by earth-and-stone walls that connect to riverside bluffs. But one can imagine that native Indians appreciated the beauty of the area as much as we do today. In what is now the state park, the two rivers drop off Highland Rim Plateau into the Nashville Basin, their waters pouring forth over big falls beside steep bluffs before meeting at the southern end of the park. Trails course through the area and along the wall of the ceremonial site. A cool, shady campground on the banks of the Duck River makes this an ideal retreat during the dog days of summer.

Enter the state park then cross the narrow bridge over the Duck River to reach the campground entrance station. Head into a very dense deciduous forest with a thick understory. Three loops spur off the main campground road, but the pretty forest is so dense that it makes the 51-site camping area seem very intimate. Paved campsite pull-ins spur off the main campground road. The thick understory of brush and small trees offers the maximum in campsite privacy, which is further enhanced by the campsites' being well separated. The ground is mostly level and in places may be prone to ponding after a big storm. Each of the three loops heads toward the Duck River. Some sites on each loop have obscured views of the water as it flows toward Bluehole Falls, which is audible from the lower part of the campground. Two modern bathhouses serve the three loops.

Although all the campsites have hookups, the campground does not resemble an RV dealership. The Old Stone Fort attracts many families and campers of

## RATINGS

Beauty: ✿ ✿ ✿ ✿
Privacy: ✿ ✿ ✿ ✿ ✿
Spaciousness: ✿ ✿ ✿ ✿
Quiet: ✿ ✿ ✿ ✿
Security: ✿ ✿ ✿
Cleanliness: ✿ ✿ ✿ ✿

all stripes. Tenters dominate the scene in summer, and RVs have a stronger presence in the cooler months, though the campground as a whole is quiet in winter. The Old Stone Fort fills only on summer weekend holidays, and with the cool, deep woods it never gets an overcrowded feel no matter the time of year. So pitch your tent and explore the Old Stone Fort.

The Old Stone Fort was never a fort in the defensive sense. Early Tennessee settlers gave it that name. Archeologists have determined that the walls delineated a ceremonial site, an enclosure built and rebuilt over a 400-year period from 30 AD to 430 AD. River cliffs served as walls as well. At the entrance to the Old Stone Fort is a museum, which is staffed every day and offers insight into the daily life of the native Indians who built the Old Stone Fort. There are ranger-led programs on summer weekends. View the exhibits inside, then tour the site. The Wall Trail makes a 1.25-mile loop along the walls and cliffs that encircle the 50-acre ceremonial site. Smaller side paths lead past the park's three major falls. Bluehole Falls and Big Falls are on the Duck River, and Step Falls is on the Little Duck River, adding natural beauty to the historic setting. These rivers also offer fishing for bream and bass.

In later days, settlers saw the falls as a source of power, and many dams were built and washed away, providing energy for sawmills, paper mills, and gristmills. Today, one dam still stands on the Duck River above Bluehole Falls and is accessible via a trail from the campground. Another short nature trail loops through the woods from near the campground entrance station. Other, wilder trails in the park are the Backbone, Little Duck Loop, and Old River Channel trails. These all spur off the Wall Trail and work through the tableland between the confluence of the two rivers. The confluence of history, beauty, and high-quality camping makes the Old Stone Fort a no-brainer for tent campers interested in exploring Tennessee.

## KEY INFORMATION

| | |
|---|---|
| **ADDRESS:** | Route 7, Box 7400 Manchester, TN 37355 |
| **OPERATED BY:** | Tennessee State Parks |
| **INFORMATION:** | (931) 723-5073; www.tnstateparks.com |
| **OPEN:** | Year-round |
| **SITES:** | 51 |
| **EACH SITE HAS:** | Picnic table, electricity, upright grill |
| **ASSIGNMENT:** | First come, first served; no reservations |
| **REGISTRATION:** | Ranger will come by to register you |
| **FACILITIES:** | Hot showers, pay phone |
| **PARKING:** | At campsites only |
| **FEE:** | Tents $15.50 per night; RVs $17.50 per night |
| **ELEVATION:** | 1,000 feet |
| **RESTRICTIONS:** | Pets: On 6-foot leash only |
| | Fires: In fire rings only |
| | Alcohol: Prohibited |
| | Vehicles: None |
| | Other: Maximum 14-day stay |

# MAP

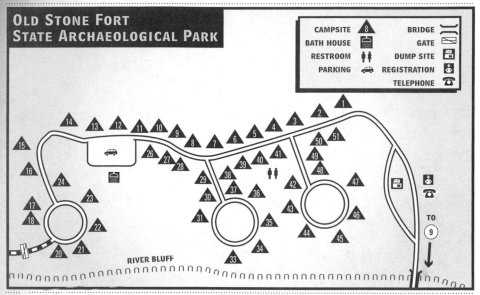

## OLD STONE FORT STATE ARCHAEOLOGICAL PARK

| | | | |
|---|---|---|---|
| CAMPSITE | ▲8 | BRIDGE | |
| BATH HOUSE | | GATE | |
| RESTROOM | | DUMP SITE | |
| PARKING | | REGISTRATION | |
| | | TELEPHONE | |

RIVER BLUFF

TO 9

# GETTING THERE

From Exit 111 on I-24 near Manchester, take TN 55 west 1 mile to US 41. Turn right and head north on US 41 through Manchester 2 miles to Old Stone Fort Archeological State Park, which will be on your left.

# PINEY

**I** **THINK 384 IS A SCARY NUMBER.** At least when you are talking about the number of campsites in a campground. This usually spells an overcrowded city of RVs, congestion, mayhem, and all the things you are trying to escape. Piney, however, bucks the trend. This getaway on the southern side of Land Between The Lakes has two loops catering to tent campers and a third loop that is a good electrical option. The campground is really well run. Add in the recreational opportunities—boating, hiking, fishing, and historical study, and you have a high-quality destination that tent campers can enjoy.

Pass the entrance kiosk to enter the campground. There are a total of eight loops, but tent campers need be concerned with only three of them. Dismiss Chestnut, Shortleaf, Dogwood, Persimmon, and Loblolly loops. The tents used there are square and metal, have wheels, and have TV antennas sticking out of them. Tent campers who like electricity should head to the Black Oak Loop. There will be pop-up campers and such here, but so there will also be tent campers. Black Oak is on a peninsula jutting into Kentucky Lake and has 92 campsites spread out along three loops. Thirty or so sites enjoy lake frontage, where campers pull up their boats. Some of this frontage is on a small lake cove, as opposed to the main lake. A hickory and oak woodland shades the widely separated sites. The large campsites have been leveled, but scant understory undermines campsite privacy. Small, wet-weather drainages break up the terrain. A grassy area lies between the camping area and a swimmer's beach. One of the two bathhouses has showers.

The Virginia and Sweetgum loops do not have electricity and thus are the realm of tent campers. Sweetgum has 34 sites and is entered via a loop shaded by sweetgum, oaks, and cedars. A couple of small

> *Don't let the size of this place scare you. Two good loops cater to tent campers.*

## RATINGS

Beauty: ☆ ☆ ☆ ☆
Privacy: ☆ ☆ ☆
Spaciousness: ☆ ☆ ☆
Quiet: ☆ ☆ ☆ ☆
Security: ☆ ☆ ☆ ☆ ☆
Cleanliness: ☆ ☆ ☆ ☆ ☆

## KEY INFORMATION

**ADDRESS:** 100 Van Morgan
Drive
Golden Pond, KY
42211

**OPERATED BY:** Forest Service

**INFORMATION:** (800) LBL-7077;
www.lbl.com

**OPEN:** March–November

**SITES:** 384

**EACH SITE HAS:** Picnic table, fire
grate, lantern post
(Virginia and
Sweetgum loops);
electricity, picnic
table, fire grate
(Black Oak Loop)

**ASSIGNMENT:** First come, first
served; no
reservations

**REGISTRATION:** At campground
kiosk

**FACILITIES:** Hot showers, water
spigots, pay phone,
camp store

**PARKING:** At campsites only

**FEE:** $12 per night
spring and fall;
add $3 per night
for electricity at
Black Oak Loop;
$13 per night dur-
ing summer

**ELEVATION:** 360 feet

**RESTRICTIONS:** Pets: On 6-foot
leash only
Fires: In fire rings
only
Alcohol: At camp-
sites only
Vehicles: 1
wheeled camping
vehicle per site
Other: Maximum
21-day stay

crossroads have campsites. Most sites at the beginning are inside the loop; swing by the lake to find some fine sites overlooking the water, which is about 30 feet away. The end of the loop has some decent sites that are a little close together. The Virginia Loop has 23 sites shaded by pines and oaks. The loop descends toward the water. The six waterside sites are some of the best in the entire campground. The other sites here a little too cramped for my taste. The end of the loop has ultrashady sites good for a hot summer afternoon. Water spigots are strategically situated throughout both loops, and a fully equipped bathhouse serves both loops. Locals are the primary tent campers, which is a good sign. Piney generally fills on summer holiday weekends. Other than that, you should have no trouble getting a site. A camp store has most supplies you'll need.

Now, what to do? The campground roads are great for biking, and bikes are available for rent from the camp store. Better yet, bring your own two-wheeler. Or go boating in Kentucky Lake and fish. Or fish without a boat at Catfish Pond. Or dip yourself in the water at the swimming beach. Hikers have the Fort Henry Trail system to tackle. There are 26 miles of paths here, and you can actually trace U. S. Grant's movements between Fort Henry and nearby Fort Donelson. These forts were the sites of the first Civil War attacks on the river routes of what was then the West. A Fort Henry Trail map reveals numerous loops. The Piney Trail leads from near the campground into this trail network.

Fort Donelson, just a few miles away on the Cumberland River, is a national battlefield and is where U. S. Grant's star first rose. You can tour the battlefield by walking 7 miles of interpretive trails or by driving along the battlefield road. Check out the river battery's big guns and the still-standing Dover Hotel, where the losing side surrendered. At Piney Campground you won't surrender to boredom or crowds, just to the joy of a good tent-camping destination.

# MAP

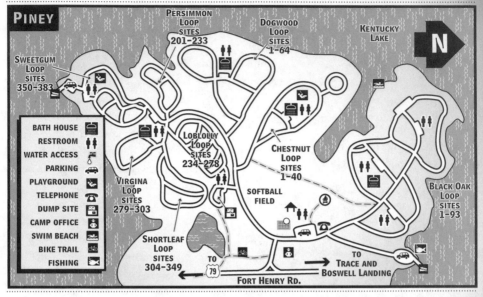

## GETTING THERE

From Dover, head 12 miles west on US 79 to Fort Henry Road. Turn right onto Fort Henry Road and follow it 2.3 miles to the campground, which will be on your left.

# RAGLAND BOTTOMS

> *Ragland Bottoms offers two types of tent sites on Center Hill Lake.*

**T**HE CANEY FORK RIVER FLOWS WEST through rugged terrain and is dammed as Center Hill Lake, where jumbled steep hills form the water's backdrop. This setting makes for some great Volunteer State scenery. Luckily for us, the Army Corps of Engineers found some land level enough— with some site work—to put in a high-quality campground with waterfront tent sites, some hillside tent sites, and camps more suited for RVs but that would nevertheless serve tent campers. And being on a lake as pretty as Center Hill makes Ragland Bottoms Campground an even better place.

The campground has several distinctly different areas in which to overnight. The first area contains sites 1 through 20. These are fully developed water and electric campsites that are close to the lake and designed for RVs. Some of the sites are pull-through. Yes, they are close to the water, but they are also a little too close to each other. There is a small playground and a bathhouse here. The next area, with sites 21 through 30, is also beside the lake and is very desirable for tent campers. These sites are walk-in tent sites set on a shaded hill that leads down to the lake. But the sites themselves are well built and level. Some of these campsites are so close to the walk-in parking area as to barely qualify as walk-in tent sites. The ones closest to the water are snapped up first, even though they are farthest from the parking area. The understory is mostly grass, which cuts down on campsite privacy, but these are the best sites for tent campers here. These sites have water and electricity and thus are a little more expensive than most walk-in tent sites.

The next area has campsites 31 through 40. These are purely RV sites, which are open to the sun and too close to one another; a tent camper wouldn't be caught dead here unless they were borrowing a cup of sugar

## RATINGS

Beauty: ☆ ☆ ☆
Privacy: ☆ ☆ ☆
Spaciousness: ☆ ☆ ☆ ☆
Quiet: ☆ ☆ ☆ ☆
Security: ☆ ☆ ☆ ☆ ☆
Cleanliness: ☆ ☆ ☆ ☆

from their big-rig neighbor. Farther up the hill and farthest from the lake are campsites 42 through 57. These primitive camps are shaded, with a grassy understory. They have been cut into the hillside and are a little small, but I wouldn't be disappointed to stay in one. Of special note to those who like solitude is campsite 55. There is a bathhouse up here serving this area that is the last to fill. Ye Old Red Post Nature Trail spurs off this loop. A slate walkway leads to a spring. Begin the loop portion of the trail beyond the spring by rounding a knob nearly encircled by Center Hill Lake. It is obvious that this part of DeKalb County is nothing but steep hills and valleys with very little level land around. Ironically, some of the most level and fertile land, including Ragland Bottoms, was submerged when Center Hill Lake was filled. Within this steep terrain a stone arch is visible through the trees. This arch is a good 30 feet across and 20 feet high and gives the appearance of a giant window carved in a rock. It is hard to get a good view because the terrain is just too steep to allow one to get very close.

Nature trail aside, most recreation revolves around Center Hill Lake. Ragland Bottoms has a day-use area with a boat ramp. It also has a swimming beach, which is popular with campers and day users. The large picnic area and picnic shelter add to the scenery. And that shelter could come in handy on a rainy day. Boaters will have an advantage because they can tour this beautiful lake and choose whether to fish, water-ski, or just enjoy the sights that make DeKalb County, and especially Ragland Bottoms, a great place to visit.

## KEY INFORMATION

| | |
|---|---|
| **ADDRESS:** | Center Hill Lake, 158 Resource Lane Lancaster, TN 38569 |
| **OPERATED BY:** | Army Corps of Engineers |
| **INFORMATION:** | (931) 858-3125; www.lrn.usace.army.mil |
| **OPEN:** | Mid-April–mid-October |
| **SITES:** | 55 |
| **EACH SITE HAS:** | Picnic table, fire, ring; some also have water and electricity |
| **ASSIGNMENT:** | First come, first served; reservations available |
| **REGISTRATION:** | At campground entrance booth |
| **FACILITIES:** | Hot showers, flush toilets, water spigots |
| **PARKING:** | At campsites and walk-in areas |
| **FEE:** | $14 per night tent sites, $18 per night tent sites with electricity, $20 other sites |
| **ELEVATION:** | 750 feet |
| **RESTRICTIONS:** | Pets: On leash only Fires: In fire rings only Alcohol: At campsites only Vehicles: 2 vehicles per site Other: Maximum 14-day stay in a 30-day period |

## MAP

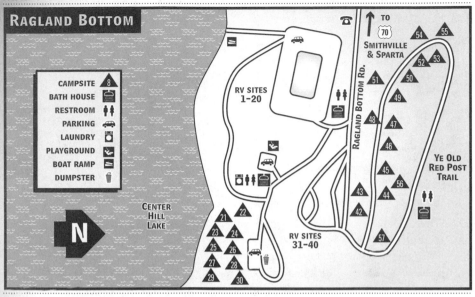

### GETTING THERE

From Smithville, take US 70 east 7 miles to Ragland Bottom Road. Ragland Bottom Road is 1 mile beyond Sligo Bridge. Turn left onto Ragland Bottom Road and follow it to the campground.

# ROCK ISLAND
# STATE PARK

**T**HESE DAYS, THE HAND OF MAN is often seen as a destructive force in nature. Here at Rock Island State Park, human forces unintentionally created what many Tennesseans, including me, consider to be the state's prettiest waterfall. Here's the story: In 1915 Tennessee Electric Power Company dammed the Caney Fork River. This dam backed up the Caney Fork and the nearby Collins River, creating Great Falls Lake. This raising of the water level forced water from the Collins River through caves that emerged on a rock face of the Caney Fork River. Since then, and to this day, water courses through the caves then makes a 300-foot-wide, 80-foot drop over a rock bluff into the Caney Fork River. This drop is known as Twin Falls. Great Falls, the lake's namesake, is actually a different scenic cascade within the park boundaries. This watery beauty is only part of the picture, however. A tent-only camping loop, trails, swimming beaches, and more make Rock Island State Park a great destination.

> *Rock Island packs an enormous amount of beauty into its boundaries.*

Let's start with the campground. Pass the park office and turn left into the tent loop. The gravel road passes beside a fully equipped bathhouse then enters shady wood of pine and cedar. This shade minimizes understory. The campsites are average in size and are evenly spaced. Although this is a designated tenter's loop, each site has water and electricity. Some campsites stretch out along the auto turnaround: these are the biggest and best sites.

The main campground has a trading post and hosts both tent and RV campers. Steep bluffs drop off the edges of the camping area. Paved pull-ins beneath the pines and mixed hardwoods attract RVs. The last part of the campground, starting with site 31, is more attractive to tent campers. Here the sites are spread far apart on the outside of the road, overlooking wooded drop-offs. The forest is thicker here, creating more

## RATINGS

Beauty: ☆ ☆ ☆ ☆
Privacy: ☆ ☆ ☆
Spaciousness: ☆ ☆ ☆
Quiet: ☆ ☆ ☆
Security: ☆ ☆ ☆ ☆ ☆
Cleanliness: ☆ ☆ ☆ ☆ ☆

## KEY INFORMATION

**ADDRESS:** 82 Beach Road Rock Island, TN 38581

**OPERATED BY:** Tennessee State Parks

**INFORMATION:** (931) 686-2471; www.tnstateparks.com

**OPEN:** Year-round

**SITES:** 60

**EACH SITE HAS:** Picnic table, fire ring, water, electricity, upright grills

**ASSIGNMENT:** First come, first served, and by reservation

**REGISTRATION:** At campground check-in station

**FACILITIES:** Hot showers, flush toilets, telephone

**PARKING:** At campsites only

**FEE:** Tent $15.50 per night; RV $17.50 per night

**ELEVATION:** 950 feet

**RESTRICTIONS:** Pets: On 6-foot leash only
Fires: In fire rings only
Alcohol: Prohibited
Vehicles: None
Other: Maximum 14-day stay

campsite privacy. Two bathhouses and a pavilion and playground serve the main campground. Tent campers will want to try the tent loop first, then this camping area. Rock Island fills only on summer holiday weekends, so getting a site is not a problem, but campsite reservations are available here, unlike at most Tennessee state parks.

Everybody loves to visit the falls here. Twin Falls Overlook is on the far side of the Caney Fork River from the campground. Cross the Great Falls Dam on the way to the overlook. Many canoers and kayakers use the Sand Bar Launch Ramp to paddle to Twin Falls, which looks enormous from the bottom. Mother Nature didn't need any help with the swimming facilities at Rock Island. There is a natural sand beach just below the boat ramp. Here swimmers bask in the cool waters of the Caney Fork River while enjoying the setting—clear, green waters against a tall rock bluff—a natural pool that makes any man-made swimming pool look bad. Others campers rock-hop and swim below Great Falls. Trails offer another way to see the park. The Collins River Nature Trail makes a loop through the land between the Collins and Caney Fork rivers. The Eagle Trail leaves directly from the campground and leads down to the banks of the Caney Fork. There is even a short mountain bike trail.

Rock Island State Park borders the uppermost reaches of Center Hill Lake. Boaters can take off from the park to fish and explore the lake, or use the boat ramp to try their luck on the lower Collins River. Game players can use the tennis, basketball, and volleyball courts after checking out equipment free of charge at the ranger station. The rangers at Rock Island pride themselves on their nature programs. There is a full-time park naturalist year-round and an additional one on staff in summer. Wood walks, cave trips, canoe trips, bird walks, and more keep the kids busy and help adults learn more about the beauty here, whether the work of nature or man.

# MAP

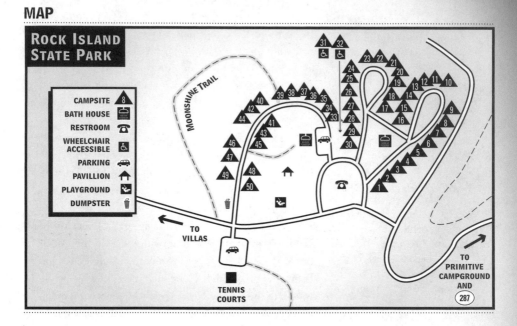

**ROCK ISLAND STATE PARK**

| | |
|---|---|
| CAMPSITE | △ 8 |
| BATH HOUSE | |
| RESTROOM | ☎ |
| WHEELCHAIR ACCESSIBLE | ♿ |
| PARKING | 🚐 |
| PAVILLION | 🏠 |
| PLAYGROUND | |
| DUMPSTER | 🗑 |

MOONSHINE TRAIL

TO VILLAS

TENNIS COURTS

TO PRIMITIVE CAMPGROUND AND
287

## GETTING THERE

From Smithville, at the junction with US 70, take TN 56 south 9.5 miles to TN 287. Turn left onto TN 287 north and take it 10.5 miles to the state park entrance, which will be on your left.

# RUSHING CREEK

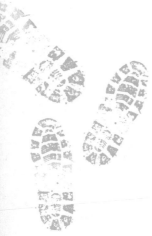

> *The name doesn't do this relaxing campground justice.*

I HAVE ENJOYED **RUSHING CREEK** in spring, summer, and fall. Suffice it to say you can't go wrong here. Spring offers the promise of renewal as plants sprout and animals awaken. Summer is ideal for water fun on Kentucky Lake. Fall is the time to enjoy land-based recreational opportunities like hiking. Campers can enjoy other nearby attractions no matter the season. Rushing Creek campground has the aura of an old-time camp but with showers. It has a relaxed feel to it, yet there is plenty to do nearby.

Let's start with the campground. Drop down to the shores of Kentucky Lake to come to the pay station. There is a campground host nearby from March through October. Continue straight and follow a gravel road toward the lake, passing a bathhouse with showers. To the left is a large picnic shelter in a grassy waterside field. To the right are three shady sites beneath oak trees. These sites feature awesome lake views. Return to the pay station and a loop heads to the right, up a small hollow. Oaks, hickories, cedars, and sycamore trees shade these 12 average-sized camps that have a grassy understory. There are several sites that are secluded because of their distance from one another. The final site has electricity; it's the only one in the campground that does. There is a water spigot near this site.

Another road leaves left from the pay station, up the hollow of an intermittent stream to well-shaded sites. Two small bridges span the stream beside a small field. The loop road rises slightly, but the sites have been leveled with landscaping timbers. Two other sites lie along a dead-end road and are so far from the others you won't see another camper unless you want to. Jones Creek Camping Area is nearby. You passed the turn for it just before reaching Rushing Creek. Follow the gravel road down to a flat beside Kentucky Lake.

## RATINGS

Beauty: ✪ ✪ ✪ ✪
Privacy: ✪ ✪ ✪ ✪
Spaciousness: ✪ ✪ ✪ ✪
Quiet: ✪ ✪ ✪ ✪
Security: ✪ ✪ ✪ ✪
Cleanliness: ✪ ✪ ✪ ✪

Fourteen campsites, not numbered but each with a picnic table and a fire ring, are spaced along an intermittent streambed. A picnic shelter stands on a hill nearby and is equipped with a vault toilet; it has no water but offers the maximum in solitude. There is a boat ramp near the camping area.

Rushing Creek will only fill on summer holiday weekends. Summer weekends are the most crowded. Solitude is guaranteed in winter. The bathhouse showers are closed from November through February.

Immediate obvious recreation is centered on Kentucky Lake. Boaters will launch from the camp ramp. Anglers can be seen fishing from shore. Swimmers enjoy the cove that opens to the main body of the lake. A playground with basketball hoops and badminton nets is located near the campground host. The field adjacent to the lake invites kites and ballgames.

If you want to roam with a purpose, take the Walker Line Trail to the North–South Trail, which stretches 60 miles, running the length of Land Between The Lakes. You can walk or drive to The Homeplace-1850. This is a working 19th-century farm where interpreters in period clothing enact the daily lives of settlers from the 1850s. There are 16 original and restored structures from the Land Between The Lakes area on this farm. Just across the road from The Homeplace-1850 is the Buffalo Range and Trail. Buffalo live on this fenced range just as they lived in this section of Tennessee long ago. North of Rushing Creek, just over the Kentucky state line, is the Golden Pond Visitor Center and Planetarium. It has programs that look to the heavens and offers star-observation sessions. Also nearby is the Elk and Bison Prairie. This is a restored "barren," a habitat once favored by elk and buffalo. You can take an auto tour of this wildlife-rich locale. Actually, the whole of Land Between The Lakes is rich with outdoor opportunities of all kinds.

## KEY INFORMATION

| | |
|---|---|
| **ADDRESS:** | 100 Van Morgan Drive Golden Pond, KY 42211 |
| **OPERATED BY:** | Forest Service |
| **INFORMATION:** | (270) 924-2000; www.lbl.org |
| **OPEN:** | Year-round |
| **SITES:** | 40 |
| **EACH SITE HAS:** | Picnic table, fire grate |
| **ASSIGNMENT:** | First come, first served; no reservations |
| **REGISTRATION:** | March–October register with host ; November–February self-registration on-site |
| **FACILITIES:** | Hot showers, water spigots March–October; vault toilets November–February |
| **PARKING:** | At campsites only |
| **FEE:** | $9 per night March–October; $8 per night November–February |
| **ELEVATION:** | 360 feet |
| **RESTRICTIONS:** | Pets: On 6-foot leash only Fires: In fire rings only Alcohol: At campsites only Vehicles: 15-mph campground speed limit Other: Maximum 21-day stay |

## MAP

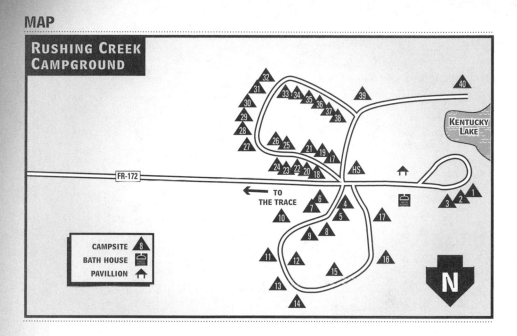

**RUSHING CREEK CAMPGROUND**

KENTUCKY LAKE

FR-172

TO THE TRACE

CAMPSITE
BATH HOUSE
PAVILLION

N

## GETTING THERE

From Dover, head 5 miles south on US 79 to access the Trace. Turn right on the Trace and drive 16.5 miles north to Forest Road 172 and follow it to dead-end at the campground.

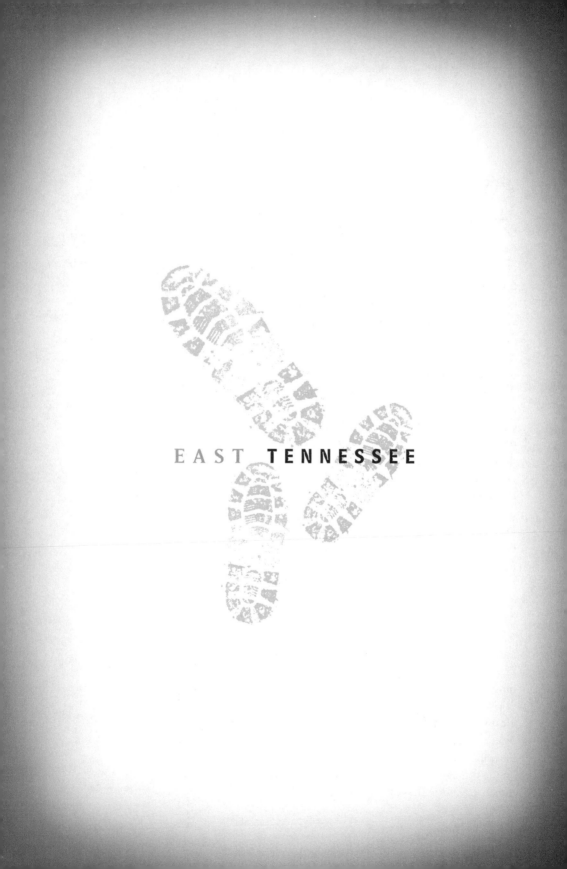

EAST TENNESSEE

# ABRAMS CREEK

**C**AMPERS DON'T JUST STUMBLE into this well-kept secret, hidden at the end of a gravel road off a meandering valley road. But those who find it make it worth their time. Located at the extreme western edge of the Smokies, Abrams Creek Campground may be off the beaten tourist path, but nearby there are plenty of footpaths, as well as a few other activities. Located in a wooded flat along a tranquil section of Abrams Creek, this intimate campground provides a relaxing setting not found in most national park campgrounds. The 16 sites are usually filled only on weekends and holidays. The place seems nearly deserted on lazy summer weekdays. About half the sites are creekside, but all are well shaded. If relaxing under a towering white pine in a quiet woodland beside a cool mountain stream is your pleasure, this is the campground for you. This place really feels like an escape from civilization. Since it is in the park's lowlands, this campground can be fairly warm, if not downright hot, in the summer. But no matter how hot it gets during the day, you can always expect it to cool down in the evening. A water fountain and cold, running water, situated in the middle of the campground, are there to slake your thirst and let you wash up.

The creek and campground were named after Old Abram, the Cherokee chief of the town of Chilhowee, which was located at the confluence of Abrams Creek and the Little Tennessee River. Since it was dammed the "Little T" has been called Chilhowee Lake. Spanning 1,747 acres, it is 9 miles long and only a mile wide at its widest point. A boat launch is conveniently located on US 129 near the Foothills Parkway, 7 miles from the campground, and anglers will find trout, bass, bluegill, and catfish awaiting their hook and line. Don't let the campground's low elevation make you underestimate the ruggedness of this country. Between the

> *Abrams Creek Campground offers national park–level beauty and recreational opportunities in an off-the-beaten-path atmosphere.*

## RATINGS

Beauty: ☆ ☆ ☆ ☆ ☆
Site Privacy: ☆ ☆ ☆
Site Spaciousness: ☆ ☆ ☆
Quiet: ☆ ☆ ☆ ☆ ☆
Security: ☆ ☆ ☆ ☆
Cleanliness: ☆ ☆ ☆ ☆ ☆

**ADDRESS:** 6537 Abrams Creek Road
Tallassee, TN 37878

**OPERATED BY:** Great Smoky Mountains National Park

**INFORMATION:** (423) 436-1200; www.nps.gov/grsm

**OPEN:** Mid-March–October

**SITES:** 16

**EACH SITE HAS:** Picnic table, fire pit, lantern post

**ASSIGNMENT:** First come, first served; no reservations

**REGISTRATION:** Self registration on site

**FACILITIES:** Flush toilets, cold running water

**PARKING:** At individual sites

**FEE:** $12 per night

**ELEVATION:** 1,125 feet

**RESTRICTIONS:** Pets: On leash only
Fires: In fire pits only
Alcohol: At campsite only
Vehicles: Small trailers up to 12 feet; no RV hookups
Other: Maximum 7-day stay

sharp, wooded ridges flow twisting streams overgrown with rhododendron, where black bear, deer, and other fauna forage for their sustenance. Within this terrain a fine trail system offers pleasant hiking. And for those in a walking frame of mind, the Cooper Road Trail, which starts at the back of the campground, is convenient. Once on the Cooper Road Trail, you can make a 7.5-mile loop hike. This will give you a good taste of the pine and oak woods within this area of the park. Combining the Little Bottoms, Hannah Mountain, and Rabbit Creek trails, you will see the Abrams Creek Gorge and a couple of old homesites and pass three backcountry campsites. The loop ends at the Abrams Creek Ranger Station near the campground. If you are feeling really aggressive, climb Pine Mountain. It's 2 miles up the Rabbit Creek Trail, starting near the ranger station. Cross Abrams Creek on a foot log with a handrail, pass the old homesite on your left, then start climbing. A semicircle of stones marks the trail's high point, where Chilhowee Mountain can be seen to the north. On the way back down, see if you can spot the ranger station between the trees.

The 10-mile round-trip walk to Abrams Falls is a rewarding hike to a popular destination, but few make the trip from Abrams Campground. To get to the falls, walk a mile on Cooper Road, turn onto the Little Bottoms Trail, and continue to follow Abrams Creek to the falls. The wide rush of Abrams Creek drops into a large plunge pool, where hot hikers often take a dip in the cool mountain water. In late spring this route is brightened by the pink and white blooms of the ubiquitous mountain laurel.

Downstream, a long quiet pool abuts the campground, enticing its share of swimmers, tubers, and anglers alike. Rainbow trout inhabit these waters, and since this is in the park's lowlands, this park stream is one of the few that includes feisty rock bass and their larger cousin, the smallmouth bass. A Tennessee state fishing license is required, but the license allows anglers to fish park waters in both Tennessee and North Carolina.

# MAP

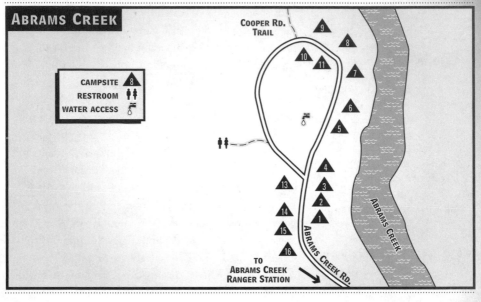

**ABRAMS CREEK**

COOPER RD.
TRAIL

| | |
|---|---|
| CAMPSITE | ▲8 |
| RESTROOM | 👫 |
| WATER ACCESS | 🚰 |

9

8

10

11

7

6

5

4

13

3

2

14

1

15

16

TO
ABRAMS CREEK
RANGER STATION

ABRAMS CREEK RD.

ABRAMS CREEK

## GETTING THERE

From Maryville, Tennessee, drive south on US 129, reaching Chilhowee Lake on your right. Turn left onto Happy Valley Road, 0.5 miles beyond the Foothills Parkway. Follow Happy Valley Road 6 miles to Abrams Creek Road. Turn right onto Abrams Creek Road and drive 1 mile to the campground, passing the ranger station on your left.

# BANDY CREEK

> *Bandy Creek Campground lies at the heart of the 100,000-acre Big South Fork National River and Recreation Area.*

**T**HE **NATIONAL PARK SERVICE** is catching on. It realizes there are two divergent groups that use campgrounds: tent campers and RVers. Here at Bandy Creek Campground, the park service has designated a tents-only loop. This is a good thing, because having a recommended campground in the Big South Fork completes the outdoor package.

Protected since 1974, the Big South Fork features wild rivers, steep gorges, thick forests, and remnants of human history atop the Cumberland Plateau. A well-developed trail system with paths leaving directly from the campground makes exploring the Big South Fork easy. There are also mountain biking, canoeing, fishing, and rafting opportunities.

Bandy Creek Campground is a large complex with a total of four camping loops. A recreational area and the park's visitor center are nearby. Loop A is the only loop reserved exclusively for tent campers. It is separated from the rest of the campground, being off to the left after you pass the campground registration booth. Most of the camping area is wooded. A few sites back up to a field and the recreation complex, which includes a swimming pool and a playground for young campers. Since Bandy Creek is atop the plateau, the forest is mixed hardwood with oaks, tulip trees, and Virginia pine. The campsites themselves are mostly open, bordered by a dense woodland. A mini-loop extends from Loop A and contains four out-of-the-way sites. Beyond the first mini-loop, campsites with paved parking areas extend on either side of the road as it rises slightly, passing one of the two most complete washhouses I've ever encountered. The buildings are designed to complement the local architecture and have a water fountain, piped water, flush toilets, showers, and even a two-basin sink for washing dishes! Farther on, the road divides and arrives at one

## RATINGS

Beauty: ☆ ☆ ☆
Privacy: ☆ ☆ ☆
Spaciousness: ☆ ☆ ☆ ☆
Quiet: ☆ ☆ ☆
Security: ☆ ☆ ☆ ☆
Cleanliness: ☆ ☆ ☆ ☆ ☆

of the two bad sites in the campground: site 32 is adjacent to the water tower; the other bad camp, site 2,
backs up to the swimming pool. As Loop A swings
around, there is a mini-loop off of it. This loop contains seven wooded sites that are the most private in
the campground. The main road passes the second
washhouse. Three other water pumps are dispersed
among the 49 well-kept sites. The rest of the campground contains 96 sites. Only Loop D, with 52 sites, is
open to both tents and RVs during the winter. The
pool is open from June to Labor Day, but the rest of
this park is ready to be explored year-round.

Hiking is very popular. Why not? Trails lace the
immediate area. The John Litton–General Slavens
Loop traverses 6 miles of surrounding countryside. It
descends to the valley where the John Litton Farm
stands, passes a large rock house, and climbs back up
to the campground via Fall Branch Falls. If you prefer
a trail with more human and natural history, take the
Oscar Blevins Loop. It is a moderate, 3.6-mile loop
that passes the Blevins Farm, some large trees, and
more of the steep bluffs that characterize the Cumberland Plateau. Another hiking option is the easy Bandy
Creek Campground loop. It is a short, 1.3-mile family
hike that offers a good introduction to the area. Want
more trails? Stop by the visitor center, and they can
point you in the right direction. If you don't feel like
walking, ride a horse. The nearby Bandy Creek Stables
offer guided rides for a fee. Water enthusiasts should
drive the short distance to Leatherwood Ford and the
Big South Fork for recreation. There the river flows
through a scenic gorge with steep cliffs soaring to the
sky. Exciting rapids and decent fishing can be found
both upstream and down. Check the visitor center for
river conditions. Mountain biking is growing in popularity, too. Obviously you won't be spending much
time relaxing at the campground. There is simply too
much to see and do. Come see the Big South Fork and
you will have spent your time well.

## KEY INFORMATION

| | |
|---|---|
| **ADDRESS:** | Route 3, Box 401 Oneida, TN 37841 |
| **OPERATED BY:** | National Park Service |
| **INFORMATION:** | (931) 879-4869 or www.nps.gov/biso; reservations, www.reservations. nps.gov or (800) 365-2267 |
| **OPEN:** | March 15– October 31; limited sites year-round |
| **SITES:** | 49 tents only, 100 other |
| **EACH SITE HAS:** | Tent pad, fire grate, picnic table, lantern post |
| **ASSIGNMENT:** | First come, first served; reserva- tions available |
| **REGISTRATION:** | Self-registration on site |
| **FACILITIES:** | Piped water, flush toilets, hot show- ers, pay phone |
| **PARKING:** | At campsites only |
| **FEE:** | $17 per night, $20 per night electric sites |
| **ELEVATION:** | 1,500 feet |
| **RESTRICTIONS:** | Pets: On a 6-foot leash only Fires: In fire grates only Alcohol: At camp- sites only Vehicles: Maxi- mum 2 vehicles per site Other: Maximum 14-day stay |

## MAP

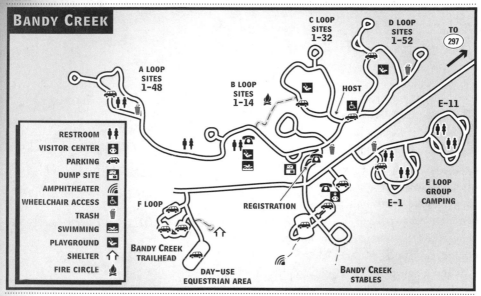

**BANDY CREEK**

A LOOP
SITES
1-48

B LOOP
SITES
1-14

C LOOP
SITES
1-32

D LOOP
SITES
1-52

TO
297

HOST

E-11

| | |
|---|---|
| RESTROOM | 👫 |
| VISITOR CENTER | |
| PARKING | 🚗 |
| DUMP SITE | |
| AMPHITHEATER | |
| WHEELCHAIR ACCESS | ♿ |
| TRASH | |
| SWIMMING | |
| PLAYGROUND | |
| SHELTER | |
| FIRE CIRCLE | 🔥 |

F LOOP

REGISTRATION

E-1

E LOOP
GROUP
CAMPING

BANDY CREEK
TRAILHEAD

DAY-USE
EQUESTRIAN AREA

BANDY CREEK
STABLES

## GETTING THERE

From Oneida, take TN 297
west 14 miles. Bandy Creek
Campground will be
on your right.

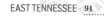

# CARDENS BLUFF

**I**F **CARDENS BLUFF WERE PRIVATE LAND** it would go for big, big bucks–the scenery is that outstanding. Luckily for us tent campers, we can overnight here for 12 bucks a shot. Tall mountains rise from the clear blue-green water of Watauga Lake. The camping area stands on a peninsula jutting into the dammed Watauga River. To make a good thing even better, the forest service has improved the campground, revamping old sites and adding walk-in tent sites and a new bathhouse with showers. To make a better thing better still, Watauga Lake offers a swimming beach, boat ramp, and hiking trails that meander through the nearby Pond Mountain Wilderness. However, Cardens Bluff is such an appealing campground that you may not even want to leave your site.

Enter the campground from TN 67. There are a few sites along the road before it makes a loop. Pass the campground host and a bathroom. A series of sites are cut into the hillside of the wooded bluff. Very few sites are directly beside the road. The dense forest screens the sites from one another and provides good shade in summer. You will soon reach the main bathhouse. This is a forest service state-of-the-art model. The wood building has separate men's and women's bathrooms with sinks and showers in them. Below to the left are several of the newest walk-in tent sites; they each have a picnic table, fire ring, lantern post, tent pad, and covered two-level food-preparation table–one level is ideal for cooking while standing. These five sites offer a mixture of sun and shade.

Just past here is an exit road with one campsite on it, campsite 12. This site offers the maximum in solitude. Another road leads to a hilltop knob where five sites perch. The main campground road curves around the peninsula and comes to a group of seven sites on a mini-peninsula of their own. They are cut into the bluff

> *Beautiful Watauga Lake is the setting for this campground that also has walk-in tent campsites.*

## RATINGS

Beauty: ✩ ✩ ✩ ✩ ✩
Privacy: ✩ ✩ ✩ ✩
Spaciousness: ✩ ✩ ✩
Quiet: ✩ ✩ ✩
Security: ✩ ✩ ✩ ✩
Cleanliness: ✩ ✩ ✩ ✩

| | |
|---|---|
| **ADDRESS:** | 4400 Unicoi Drive Unicoi, TN 37692 |
| **OPERATED BY:** | Forest Service |
| **INFORMATION:** | (423) 638-4109; www.fs.fed.us/r8/cherokee |
| **OPEN:** | Mid-April– mid-October |
| **SITES:** | 43 |
| **EACH SITE HAS:** | Picnic table, fire ring, lantern post, tent pad; some have additional cooking tables |
| **ASSIGNMENT:** | First come, first served; no reservations |
| **REGISTRATION:** | Self-registration on site |
| **FACILITIES:** | Hot showers, flush toilets, water spigots |
| **PARKING:** | At campsites only |
| **FEE:** | $12 per night |
| **ELEVATION:** | 1,990 feet |
| **RESTRICTIONS:** | Pets: On 6-foot leash only Fires: In fire rings only Alcohol: At campsites only Vehicles: Maximum 2 vehicles per site Other: Maximum 14-day stay |

and offer great lake views. Keep swinging around the hillside to reach sites on both sides of the steep hill. Attractive rock work and site leveling enhance the camps. Farther along the main loop are more roadside sites. Look for a trail leaving right that heads to four first-rate walk-in tent sites that even the most discriminating tent camper would love. Of special note is 42, which commands a view of the lake.

Such a great campground is sure to be busy. Expect the camp to fill up on nice summer weekends, and get here early if you can. You can find a site most any weekday, except during the summer holidays. There is only one shower-equipped bathhouse, but four other bathrooms are spread through the campground, as are water spigots.

At nearly 2,000 feet, Watauga Lake stays invigoratingly cool even at the height of summer. The Watauga River drains the high country of upper East Tennessee and North Carolina. This clear mountain water makes for an ultraclear lake. Just down the way is the Rat Branch boat ramp, where you can get your craft in the water and have a ball, whether you are fishing or just boating. Also down the lake is the Shooks Branch Recreation Area, which has a swimming beach. Maybe they put the swimming beach here for the Appalachian Trail (A.T.) thru-hikers since the A.T. runs right by here. If you leave south from Shook Branch on the A.T., enter the Pond Mountain Wilderness and climb to Pond Flats 4 miles distant. If you head north, the A.T. skirts the lake to reach Watauga Dam in 3 miles. The northbound hike is easier. Cardens Bluff Trail is also easy. It leaves near campsite 12 and circles around the shoreline. If you want a tough climb, head up Pond Mountain Trail. This path makes the 3.3-mile climb of Pond Mountain to a point known as Bear Stand, also in the wilderness. Pick this trail up 1.5 miles farther down TN 67 beyond the entrance to Cardens Bluff. The Watauga Point Recreation Area is only a mile down TN 67. This spot also has a swimming beach, a picnic area, and a gravel path looping through the woods.

# MAP

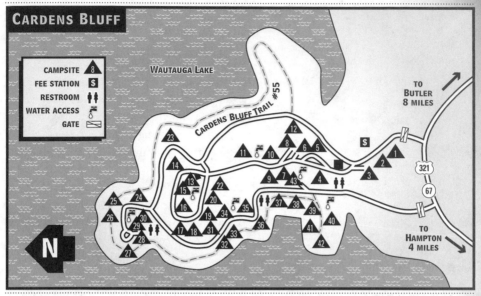

**CARDENS BLUFF**

| | |
|---|---|
| CAMPSITE | 8 |
| FEE STATION | S |
| RESTROOM | 👥 |
| WATER ACCESS | 🚰 |
| GATE | ▱ |

WAUTAUGA LAKE

CARDENS BLUFF TRAIL #55

TO BUTLER 8 MILES

321

67

TO HAMPTON 4 MILES

N

## GETTING THERE

From the junction of US 19 and US 321 in Elizabethton, head 5 miles south on US 321/US 19/TN 67 to Hampton. Here TN 67 turns left into Hampton. Follow TN 67 east 4.1 miles to the campground, on your left.

# CHILHOWEE

> *Enjoy this mountaintop campground, which has plenty of activities to keep campers busy and happy.*

**T**HE **CHILHOWEE EXPERIENCE STARTS** on the road to the campground. Forest Service Road 77 is a Forest Service–designated scenic byway that climbs 7 miles to the campground. Don't rush the trip—pull off at one of the cleared overlooks and enjoy the view of Parksville Lake below and the mountains and valleys undulating in the distance. Once you've made the pull to the top and seen the campground, it's the nearby activities that will keep you up there for a while.

This mountaintop campground is a cool retreat on hot summer days. Popular with families, many of whom return year after year, Chilhowee fills up on weekends and holidays. Although there are 25 sites with electric hookups, tent camping is the norm here; the steep drive up the mountain discourages most RVs and trailers. The campground itself is spread across three distinct areas. Loops A and B are the oldest and highest, built in the 1930s by the Civilian Conservation Corps. They are nestled beneath a hardwood forest in a dip on the mountain. Water spigots are well placed and accessible to all campers. Two comfort stations with flush toilets are available for each sex, but only Loop B has showers. A campground host keeps the area clean, safe, and secure. Loops C, D, E, and F are newer and more spacious. They are placed according to the mountainous terrain and have more ground cover for privacy beneath the piney woods. Two comfort stations serve the four loops, but only Loop F has showers. Water is easily accessible in these loops.

The third area, for overflow camping, is in an open, grassy field ringed by woods. It has one comfort station, but no shower, for the 23 overflow sites. There is one water source here. Too close together, the sites are neither spacious nor private, but campers make the most of it because of the numerous recreational opportunities nearby.

## RATINGS

**Beauty:** ✰ ✰ ✰ ✰
**Privacy:** ✰ ✰ ✰
**Spaciousness:** ✰ ✰ ✰ ✰
**Quiet:** ✰ ✰ ✰
**Security:** ✰ ✰ ✰ ✰ ✰
**Cleanliness:** ✰ ✰ ✰ ✰ ✰

Want to take a hike? You won't have to go far from camp. The Azalea Trail begins in Loop F, climbing the ridge above the campground then making a 2-mile loop back. Or keep going on the Clear Creek Trail to the northern rim of the Rock Creek Gorge Scenic Area. Benton Falls Trail starts near Lake McCamy and travels 1.6 miles to end at the 65-foot falls. Be careful: it gets steep toward the end. Bicyclists can stretch their legs, too. Pedal the Red Leaf Trail to Benton Falls or ride the Arbutus Trail. If you're quiet, you might see some wildlife. All trails are open to both bikers and hikers.

If all that exercise gets you steamed up, take a dip in 3-acre Lake McCamy. At the swimming beach on the northern end, sunbathers lie in the sun then cool off in the water. Anglers may try to catch bream and bass from the shore or toss a line from a small nonmotorized boat. Visible from the mountain along US 64 is the famed Ocoee River. For years the water was diverted from the streambed into an old wooden flume to generate power. When the flume began to leak, the water was again let loose into the Ocoee riverbed. Paddling enthusiasts realized that the long-lost rapids would be a wonderful challenge in a canoe, kayak, or raft, and the new recreational opportunity has been an economic boon to the area ever since, with paddlers coming from all over the world to test the waters. The upper Ocoee was the site of the 1996 Olympic whitewater events. Outfitters will guide you down the crashing whitewater on a hair-raising raft ride.

Also along US 64 you'll find the Scenic Spur Trail, a hiking-only venture into the heart of the Rock Creek Gorge Scenic Area. Slowly ascend the 1.7-mile footpath to see the effects of water, time, and the elements on the land. With all there is to do out there, don't forget that you have a campground to return to in the evenings.

## KEY INFORMATION

| | |
|---|---|
| ADDRESS: | Route 1, Box 348D Benton, TN 37307 |
| OPERATED BY: | Forest Service |
| INFORMATION: | (423) 338-5201; www.fs.fed.us/r8/cherokee |
| OPEN: | April–early November |
| SITES: | 88 |
| EACH SITE HAS: | Picnic table, grill, lantern post |
| ASSIGNMENT: | First come, first served; no reservations |
| REGISTRATION: | Self-registration on site |
| FACILITIES: | Flush toilets, warm showers, drinking water |
| PARKING: | At campsites only |
| FEE: | $12 per night; $15 with electricity (some are $20) |
| ELEVATION: | 2,600 feet |
| RESTRICTIONS: | Pets: On leash only Fires: In fire grates only Alcohol: Prohibited Vehicles: Do not park overnight in the day-use lot Other: Maximum 5 persons per campsite; maximum 14-day stay |

# MAP

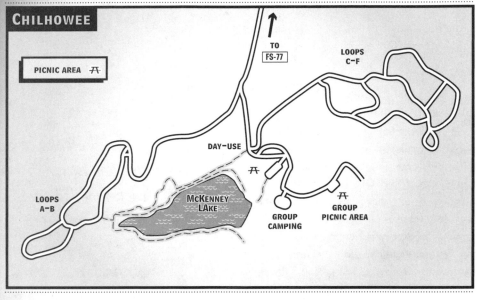

## GETTING THERE

From Cleveland, take US 64 east 12 miles to FS 77, just past the Ocoee District Ranger Station. Follow FS 77 about 7 miles. Chilhowee Campground will be on your right.

# COSBY

**S**ET ON A SLIGHT INCLINE in what once was pioneer farmland, this attractive terraced campground is surrounded on three sides by mountains. The large camping area is situated between the confluence of Rock Creek and Cosby Creek. On my trips to the area I have rarely seen Cosby Campground crowded, whereas other equally large Smokies campgrounds are sometimes cramped, noisy, and overflowing. Several loops expand the campground, and bathrooms are conveniently located throughout the site. A small store specializing in campers' supplies is located where you turn off TN 32.

Now beautifully reforested, this area is rich in Smoky Mountain history. Cosby was one of the most heavily settled areas in the Smokies before Uncle Sam began buying up land for a national park in the East. The farmland was marginal anyway, so, in order to supplement their income, Cosby residents set up moonshine stills in the remote hollows of this rugged country. As a result Cosby became known as the "moonshine capital of the world."

In remote brush-choked hollows along little streamlets, "blockaders"—as moonshiners were known—established stills. Before too long they had clear whiskey, "mountain dew," ready for consumption. Government agents, known as "revenuers," who were determined to stop the production and sale of "corn likker," battled the moonshiners throughout the hills. It is doubtful that any stills operate within the park boundaries today; however, in other areas of Cocke County someone is surely practicing the art of "feeding the furnace, stirring the mash, and judging the bead."

Its past is what makes Cosby so interesting. Trails split off in every direction, allowing campers to explore the human and natural history of this area. Follow the Lower Mount Cammerer Trail 1.5 miles to Sut-

> *Located off the principal tourist circuit, this cool, wooded campground makes an ideal base for exploring the virgin forests and high country of the Cosby–Greenbrier area.*

## RATINGS

Beauty: ✪ ✪ ✪ ✪ ✪
Privacy: ✪ ✪ ✪
Spaciousness: ✪ ✪ ✪ ✪
Quiet: ✪ ✪ ✪ ✪
Security: ✪ ✪ ✪ ✪
Cleanliness: ✪ ✪ ✪ ✪ ✪

**ADDRESS:** 107 Park Head-
quaters Road,
Gatlinburg, TN
37738

**OPERATED BY:** Great Smoky
Mountains
National Park

**INFORMATION:** (865) 436-1200;
www.nps.gov/grsm

**OPEN:** May–September

**SITES:** 175

**EACH SITE HAS:** Picnic table, fire
pit, lantern post

**ASSIGNMENT:** First come, first
served; no
reservations

**REGISTRATION:** At the hut at the
campground's
entrance

**FACILITIES:** Cold water, flush
toilets

**PARKING:** At individual sites

**FEE:** $14 per night

**ELEVATION:** 2,459 feet

**RESTRICTIONS:** Pets: On leash only
Fires: In fire pits
only
Alcohol: At camp-
sites only
Vehicles: None
Other: Maximum
7-day stay in
summer

ton Ridge Overlook. On the way to the overlook watch for signs of homesteaders from bygone days: rock walls, springs, and old chimneys. At the overlook you'll get a good lay of the land: Gabes Mountain to your east, the main crest of the Smokies to your south, the Cosby Valley below, and the hills of East Tennessee on the horizon.

Another hiking option is the Gabes Mountain Trail. Along its 6.6-mile length, this trail passes picturesque Henwallow Falls and meanders through huge old-growth hemlock and tulip trees and scattered old homesites. Turn around at the Sugar Cove backcountry campsite.

Don't forget to explore nearby Greenbrier. The 4-mile Ramsay Cascades Trail traverses virgin forest and ends at a picturesque waterfall that showers hikers with a fine mist. The Brushy Mountain Trail winds its way through several vegetation zones to an impressive view of the looming mass of Mount LeConte above and Gatlinburg below. Grapeyard Ridge Trail is the area's most historical and secluded hike. Walk old country paths along Rhododendron Creek and count the homesites amid fields slowly being obscured by the forest. At 3 miles, just before the Injun Creek backcountry campsite, look for the old tractor that made its last turn in these Smoky Mountains.

The crown jewel trek from Cosby Campground is the 6-mile hike to the restored Mount Cammerer fire tower. Built on a rock outcrop, it was formerly called "White Rock" by Tennesseans and "Sharp Top" by Carolinians. It has since been renamed Mount Cammerer, after Arno B. Cammerer, the former director of the National Park Service. Restored by a philanthropic outfit called "Friends of the Smokies," the squat, wood-and-stone tower was originally built by the Civilian Conservation Corps during the Depression. The 360-degree view is well worth the climb. To the north is the Cosby Valley and the rock cut of I-40. Mount Sterling and its fire tower are to the south. The main crest of the Smokies stands to the west, and a wave of mountains fades away on the eastern horizon.

Cosby Campground is a real winner. Where else can you set up your tent in the middle of history? In

## MAP

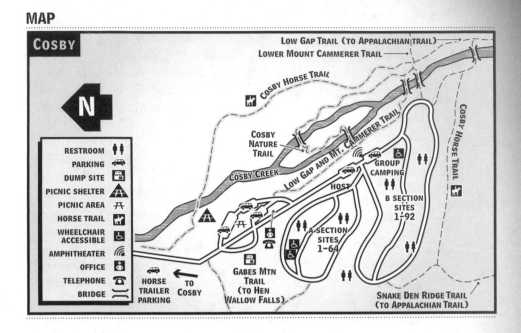

COSBY

LOW GAP TRAIL (TO APPALACHIAN TRAIL)
LOWER MOUNT CAMMERER TRAIL

COSBY HORSE TRAIL

COSBY
NATURE
TRAIL

COSBY CREEK

LOW GAP AND MT. CAMMERER TRAIL

COSBY HORSE TRAIL

GROUP
CAMPING

HOST

B SECTION
SITES
1–92

A SECTION
SITES
1–64

GABES MTN
TRAIL
(TO HEN
WALLOW FALLS)

HORSE
TRAILER
PARKING

TO
COSBY

SNAKE DEN RIDGE TRAIL
(TO APPALACHIAN TRAIL)

| | |
|---|---|
| RESTROOM | |
| PARKING | |
| DUMP SITE | |
| PICNIC SHELTER | |
| PICNIC AREA | |
| HORSE TRAIL | |
| WHEELCHAIR ACCESSIBLE | |
| AMPHITHEATER | |
| OFFICE | |
| TELEPHONE | |
| BRIDGE | |

the summer, naturalist programs in the campground amphitheater offer campers a chance to learn more about the area from rangers and other park personnel. The campground's size allows campers to set up near or away from others to achieve their perfect degree of solitude. If you are in the mood for company, however, the tourist mecca of Gatlinburg is nearby. There, you can visit an Elvis museum, see a musical revue, stock up on souvenirs, and stuff yourself with taffy.

## GETTING THERE

From Gatlinburg, take US 321 east until it comes to a T intersection with TN 32. Follow TN 32 a little over a mile, turning right into the signed Cosby section of the park. After 2.1 miles, you will arrive at the campground registration hut. The campground is just beyond the hut.

# DENNIS COVE

> *Recreational opportunities abound at every turn.*

**C**AMP HERE TO ENJOY THE DELIGHTFUL national forest that surrounds this fine campground. It can be busy on weekends, but no busier than other national forest campgrounds. There are fishing and hiking opportunities at Dennis Cove that will help you recoup some of the investment you've made in these public lands. They are, after all, yours to enjoy. The intimate campground is set in a small flat alongside Laurel Fork. A steep, sloped ridge and thickly wooded creek hem in the campground. There is no mistake, you are deep in the bosom of the Southern Appalachians. The Appalachian Trail, with its unparalleled views of Eastern mountain beauty, runs near here and is easily accessed from the campground.

As you pull into the campground, a small grassy glade is bathed in sunlight in this deeply forested cove. This area was timbered in the 1920s but has recovered nicely. A teardrop-shaped loop contains 13 of the 16 campsites. The first two sites abut the glade. Two other sites lie inside the loop, which has a grassy area of its own. The next three sites on the outside of the loop are heavily shaded by hemlock trees. Then the loop swings around to the four most popular sites, situated alongside gurgling Laurel Fork. The understory is denser here, owing to the abundance of rhododendron, which thrives in the cool, moist environs of Appalachian streams. Two more sites are widely spaced on the outside of the gravel road as it completes the loop. Hardwoods mix with a few white pines in these flat sites.

There are three other sites on the other side of the gravel road leading to the loop. These sites, large by any campground's standard, are carved out of the steep hill bordering Dennis Cove. Each site is separated by woodland from the others. If it has rained lately, as it often does here, these spots are your best bet for a dry campsite.

## RATINGS

Beauty: ☆ ☆ ☆ ☆
Privacy: ☆ ☆ ☆
Spaciousness: ☆ ☆ ☆ ☆ ☆
Quiet: ☆ ☆ ☆ ☆
Security: ☆ ☆ ☆
Cleanliness: ☆ ☆ ☆

Three water spigots are evenly dispersed about the loop. Just turn the handle and the water is yours. A small comfort station, with one flush toilet for each sex, is 100 feet off the loop away from the campground entrance. Moss growing on the stones in this area is evidence that the campground has been around a long time; however, it is revamped periodically. Before my visit, the loop road was freshly graveled and the fire rings were rebuilt.

Explore your surroundings after you've set up camp. The waterfall enthusiast has three destinations within walking distance. Walk the half mile back toward Hampton and you'll soon see a creek on the left. Follow the old 0.8-mile trail, often trod by Dennis Cove campers, up to Coon Den Falls. If you continue beyond the falls, you can access the Appalachian Trail (A.T.). Turn left and climb along White Rocks Mountain to Moreland Gap trail shelter. A little farther back down Forest Service Road 50 toward Hampton you'll find more of the A.T. Leave directly from FS 50 and follow the old railroad grade into the Laurel Fork Gorge and the Pond Mountain Wilderness. Rock outcrops and a riverine environment characterize the path to Laurel Falls. If you keep going, you'll end up in Maine.

Forest Trail 39 leaves from the campground and follows Laurel Fork into the high country. This trail crosses Laurel Fork several times as it leads upstream to Laurel Falls. The trail is popular with anglers, who match wits with the secretive brown trout that inhabit Laurel Fork. The Lacy Trap Trail, which leaves Laurel Fork in a field, leads to the A.T. and offers a great loop hike that I have enjoyed. The recreational opportunities available near Dennis Cove are limited only by your desire. The 6,000-acre Pond Mountain Wilderness is close by, as is mountain-rimmed Watauga Lake. So find some time and head on over.

## KEY INFORMATION

| | |
|---|---|
| **ADDRESS:** | 4400 Unicoi Drive Unicoi, TN 37692 |
| **OPERATED BY:** | Forest Service |
| **INFORMATION:** | (423) 638-4109; www.fs.fed.us/r8/cherokee |
| **OPEN:** | May–September |
| **SITES:** | 15 |
| **EACH SITE HAS:** | Tent pad, fire ring, lantern post, picnic table |
| **ASSIGNMENT:** | First come, first served; no reservations |
| **REGISTRATION:** | Self-registration on site |
| **FACILITIES:** | Water spigot, flush toilets |
| **PARKING:** | At campsites only |
| **FEE:** | $10 per night |
| **ELEVATION:** | 2,650 feet |
| **RESTRICTIONS:** | Pets: On 6-foot or shorter leash Fires: In fire rings only Alcohol: Prohibited Vehicles: None Other: Maximum 14-day stay |

## MAP

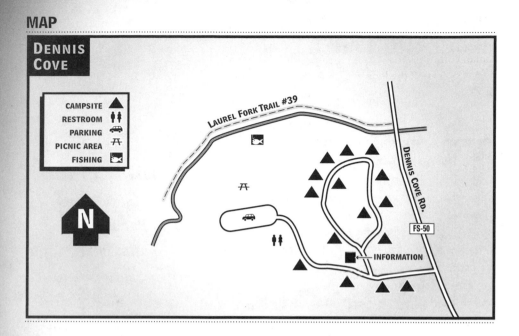

**DENNIS COVE**

CAMPSITE ▲
RESTROOM ♐♐
PARKING 🚗
PICNIC AREA 🏕
FISHING 🎣

**N**

LAUREL FORK TRAIL #39

DENNIS COVE RD.

FS-50

INFORMATION

## GETTING THERE

From Hampton, drive
0.8 miles north on US 321.
Watch carefully for the sign
with the picture of a tent on
it on the right. Turn right
there, onto the unmarked
Dennis Cove Road. Climb
away from Hampton, traveling 3.9 twisting, turning
miles. Dennis Cove Camp-
ground will be on your right.

# FOSTER FALLS RECREATION AREA

**T**HE SOUTHERN END OF THE Cumberland Plateau has some of the wildest, roughest country in Tennessee. Sheer bluffs border deep gulfs—what natives call gorges. In these gorges flow wild streams strewn with rock gardens hosting a variety of vegetation. Intermingled within this is a human history of logging and mining that has given way to the nonextractive use of nature: ecotourism.

Foster Falls Recreation Area is operated by the Tennessee Valley Authority. It offers a safe and appealing base for your camping experience in the South Cumberland Mountains. The campground is situated on a level wooded tract near Foster Falls. It features the classic loop design, only the loop is so large it seems to engulf the 26 sites spaced along it. Hardwoods give way to pines as you head toward the forested back of the loop. The umbrella magnolia is one of the campground's most interesting trees. Its leaves can reach two feet in length, causing its limbs to sag in the summer. Look for the tree along the campground entrance road and among sites 1 through 10.

The spindly, second-growth tree trunks form a light understory, but the campsites are so diffused that site privacy isn't compromised. The understory actually lends a parklike atmosphere to the campground. Foster Falls has some of the most spacious campsites I've ever seen. The large, concrete picnic tables have concrete bases to keep your feet clean when it rains. Tent pads are conspicuously absent, but there is plenty of flat terrain for pitching your tent.

The three water spigots are handy to all campsites, but the comfort station is located on one side of the loop, making a midnight bathroom run a little long for distant campers. However, this campground is rarely full, so you should be able to secure a site near the comfort station if you prefer a shorter trip. Quite often,

> *Make Foster Falls your headquarters for exploring the South Cumberland Recreation Area.*

## RATINGS

Beauty: ✩ ✩ ✩ ✩
Privacy: ✩ ✩ ✩
Spaciousness: ✩ ✩ ✩ ✩
Quiet: ✩ ✩ ✩ ✩
Security: ✩ ✩ ✩
Cleanliness: ✩ ✩ ✩

**ADDRESS:** 498 Foster Road
Sequatchie, TN
37374

**OPERATED BY:** Tennessee Valley
Authority

**INFORMATION:** (423) 942-9987 or
(800) 882-5263;
www.tva.gov

**OPEN:** Early-April–mid-
November

**SITES:** 26

**EACH SITE HAS:** Fire grate, picnic
table, lantern post

**ASSIGNMENT:** First come, first
served; no
reservations

**REGISTRATION:** Resident manager
will come by to
register you

**FACILITIES:** Water, flush toilets

**PARKING:** At campsites only

**FEE:** $14 per night

**ELEVATION:** 1,750 feet

**RESTRICTIONS:** Pets: On a 6-foot
leash only
Fires: In fire grates
only
Alcohol: Not
allowed
Vehicles: None
Other: Maximum
14-day stay

your camping companions will be rock climbers, for Foster Falls has quietly emerged as the premier rock-climbing area in the Southeast. A campground manager lives on site across from the campground entrance, providing for the security of your gear while you check out the rest of the South Cumberland Recreation Area (SCRA).

The SCRA has eight different land units, totaling over 12,000 acres, for you to enjoy. For starters, a connector trail leaves the campground to Foster Falls. Here you can take the short loop trail that leads to the base of 120-foot Foster Falls or else intersect the southern end of the Fiery Gizzard Trail and see Foster Falls from the top looking down. If you take the Fiery Gizzard Trail, you will be rewarded with views into Little Gizzard and Fiery Gizzard gulfs. Trail signs point out the rock bluffs where rock climbers have their fun. The first 2.5 miles offer many vistas and small waterfalls where side creeks plunge into the gorge below. My favorite view is from the Laurel Creek Gorge Overlook, where rock bluffs on the left meld into forested drop-offs beyond, contrasting with the flat plateau in the background.

Other must-sees in the South Cumberlands are Grundy Forest, Grundy Lakes, Savage Gulf, and the Great Stone Door. Administrators at Foster Falls will direct you to all the sights. Grundy Forest contains about 4 miles of the most feature-packed hiking you can ask for: waterfalls, rock houses, old trees, old mines, and strange rock formations. Just remember to watch where you walk, as the trails can be rough. Grundy Lakes State Park is on the National Historic Register. Once the site of mining activity, this area has seen prison labor, revolts, and the cooling down of the infamous Lone Rock coke ovens. Lone Rock Trail will lead you to all the interesting sites.

At Savage Gulf State Natural Area, three gorges converge to form a giant crow's foot. An extensive trail system connects the area's cliffs, waterfalls, sinkholes, and historic sites. The Great Stone Door is a 10-by-100-foot crack in the Big Creek Gorge that was used by Native Americans who traversed Savage Gulf. The campground at Foster Falls is pleasant enough to keep

## MAP

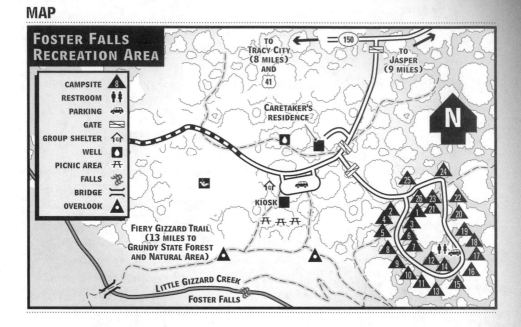

**FOSTER FALLS RECREATION AREA**

| | |
|---|---|
| CAMPSITE | 8 |
| RESTROOM | ♀♂ |
| PARKING | 🚐 |
| GATE | ▱ |
| GROUP SHELTER | 🏠 |
| WELL | ◨ |
| PICNIC AREA | 🌲 |
| FALLS | ≋ |
| BRIDGE | ≈ |
| OVERLOOK | ▲ |

TO TRACY CITY (8 MILES) AND 41

TO JASPER (9 MILES)

150

**N**

CARETAKER'S RESIDENCE

KIOSK

FIERY GIZZARD TRAIL (13 MILES TO GRUNDY STATE FOREST AND NATURAL AREA)

LITTLE GIZZARD CREEK

FOSTER FALLS

you a week or more, and that's about how long you'll need to get a good taste of the South Cumberland Recreation Area.

## GETTING THERE

From Tracy City, take US 41 south 8 miles and turn right at the sign for Foster Falls. The campground will be 0.3 miles down on your left.

# FRANKLIN STATE FOREST

*Its designation as a state forest means Franklin is little used, but its natural beauty exceeds the beauty of many state parks.*

**F**RANKLIN STATE FOREST IS ONE of those quiet, out-of-the-way places that seem to stay out of the public eye and are used only by locals. However, word is spreading about this mountain-biking and hiking mecca where the Cumberland Plateau drops sharply into Swedens Cove to form an escarpment with far-reaching views from the trail system running along its edge. Tent campers will find the campground here rustic, even down to the homemade picnic tables. The Tennessee Division of Forestry will be the first to tell you they aren't in the campground business. However, they do maintain this pretty little camp beside an unnamed lake of a few acres for those who want to explore the 7,000-acre slice of plateau country near the Alabama border.

To reach the camping area drive down gravel Lake Road and you will soon come to a solo campsite on the right side of Lake Road, all by itself near TN 156. It is in a grassy area ringed in trees, with a little gravel turnaround. This is for those who seek maximum solitude. Drive farther down the road to reach the main camping area. It is situated in a hickory-and-oak forest beside the spring-fed pond. Three separate campsites are spread along the waters, near an earthen dam. The homemade picnic tables, which add a neat rustic touch, are made from small tree trunks topped with rough-cut lumber. The sites are plenty spacious, and privacy is not much of an issue, as this campground is rarely used on weekdays and not a whole lot on weekends. Continue on the gravel road below the dam and splash over the lake outflow to reach the rest of the camping area, which is on the far side of the lake. There is a large campsite here along with a rough wooden privy.

This forest was established in 1936, then developed by the Civilian Conservation Corps after being

## RATINGS

Beauty: ☆ ☆ ☆ ☆
Privacy: ☆ ☆ ☆
Spaciousness: ☆ ☆ ☆ ☆
Quiet: ☆ ☆ ☆ ☆ ☆
Security: ☆ ☆ ☆
Cleanliness: ☆ ☆ ☆

bought from a coal operation. It is covered with miles of old roads for exploring by auto or bike. You can also use the main trail system. The campground is the trailhead for the Tom Pack Falls Trail. This trail is recommended for hiking only. It makes an approximate 2-mile loop down to the falls and back. Another trail rings the unnamed campground lake.

After you are done exploring, throw a line from your campsite and see what bites. It may be catfish, bream, or bass. Fishing is not the only activity you can enjoy directly from your tent. The entire trail system is accessible from the campground. Pump up the tires on your mountain bike and head for the rim of the Cumberland Plateau. The Swedens Cove Trail and the Fern Trail both head out from the camping area and cross TN 156 to reach the South and West Rim trails. Here, mountain bikers and hikers both cruise the path that circles the steep edge of Swedens Cove. You can gain good views into the lowlands to the southeast toward the Tennessee River and Guntersville Lake. The 6.5-mile West Rim Trail ends on TN 156, where you can park a second car to avoid backtracking. But this area is worth seeing twice. Of course most folks overlook it altogether. Grab a trail map at the ranger station, which is a log cabin just a bit north of Lake Road on TN 156.

Another nearby attraction is Russell Cave National Monument, just a few miles into Alabama, and Carter State Natural Area. Russell Cave National Monument is a preserved archeological site where native Indians lived in pre-Columbian times. History exhibits and ranger-led cave tours enhance visitors' experience.

## KEY INFORMATION

| | |
|---|---|
| **ADDRESS:** | P.O. Box 68 Winchester, TN 37398 |
| **OPERATED BY:** | Tennessee Division of Forestry |
| **INFORMATION:** | (931) 598-5507 www.state.tn.us/ agriculture/forestry |
| **OPEN:** | Year-round |
| **SITES:** | 5 |
| **EACH SITE HAS:** | Picnic table, fire ring |
| **ASSIGNMENT:** | First come, first served; no reservations |
| **REGISTRATION:** | No registration |
| **FACILITIES:** | Vault toilet; bring water |
| **PARKING:** | At campsites only |
| **FEE:** | None |
| **ELEVATION:** | 1,800 feet |
| **RESTRICTIONS:** | Pets: On 6-foot leash only Fires: In fire rings only Alcohol: Prohibited Vehicles: Maximum 2 vehicles per site Other: Maximum 14-day stay |

## MAP

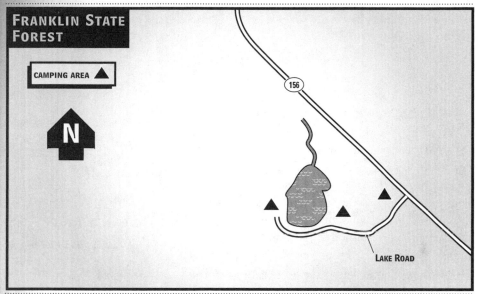

FRANKLIN STATE FOREST

CAMPING AREA ▲

N

156

LAKE ROAD

## GETTING THERE

From downtown South
Pittsburg, 2 miles south of
Exit 152 on I-24, take
TN 156 north 16.7 miles to
Lake Road. Make a hard left
turn and follow Lake Road
0.7 miles to the main
camping area.

# FROZEN HEAD STATE PARK

**F**ROZEN HEAD IS A LITTLE-KNOWN jewel of a
state park tucked away in the Cumberland
Mountains, a mountain range west of the Smokies. Steep forested peaks and deep valleys diffused with
rock formations characterize this state park that was
settled in the early 1800s by simple farmers. But the
land, so rich in coal and timber resources, was sold to
the state for the establishment of the now-infamous
Brushy Mountain State Prison, and the resources were
extracted using prison labor. The logging era ended in
the 1920s, and Frozen Head was declared a forest
reserve. The Civilian Conservation Corps came in and
established many of the trails that are in use today. A
plaque at the main trailhead memorializes those who
lost their lives developing the area. This is an ideal
park for active people who like a small campground
but want plenty of activities all within walking distance
of the campground.

Frozen Head's campground is known as Big Cove
Camping Area. A figure-eight loop contains 19 sites
that border Big Cove Branch and Flat Fork Creek.
Big Cove backs up to Bird Mountain and has a minor
slope. The sites have been leveled and are set amid
large boulders that came to rest untold eons ago after
falling from Bird Mountain. The gray boulders strewn
about give it a distinctive Cumberland Mountains
feel. Second-growth hardwoods provide ample shade,
and the dogwood and hemlock understory allow some
privacy for campers. A covered shed contains split firewood for campers to use. The bathhouse is close to all,
being in the middle of the campground. Single-sex hot
showers and flush toilets are well maintained. Two spigots provide drinking water for the small campground.

Some sites are close together, but all provide
enough room to spread out your gear. Two group sites
are available and can be reserved. Ten sites allow tent

> *Stay at Frozen Head
> and explore the water-
> falls, rock shelters, and
> mountaintop caprocks
> of the Cumberland
> Mountains.*

## RATINGS

Beauty: ☆ ☆ ☆ ☆ ☆
Privacy: ☆ ☆ ☆
Spaciousness: ☆ ☆ ☆ ☆
Quiet: ☆ ☆ ☆ ☆ ☆
Security: ☆ ☆ ☆ ☆ ☆
Cleanliness: ☆ ☆ ☆ ☆ ☆

## KEY INFORMATION

**ADDRESS:** 964 Flat Fork Road Wartburg, TN 37887

**OPERATED BY:** Tennessee State Parks

**INFORMATION:** (423) 346-3318; www.tnstateparks.com

**OPEN:** Mid-March– mid-November

**SITES:** 20

**EACH SITE HAS:** Picnic table, fire grate with grill, lantern post, firewood

**ASSIGNMENT:** First come, first served; no reservations

**REGISTRATION:** At visitor center

**FACILITIES:** Water, flush toilets, hot showers

**PARKING:** At campsites only

**FEE:** $13 per night mid-March–October, $11 per night rest of year

**ELEVATION:** 1,500 feet

**RESTRICTIONS:** Pets: On leash only Fires: In fire grates only Alcohol: Not allowed Vehicles: A narrow bridge crossing limits trailers to 16 feet Other: Maximum 14-day stay

and trailer camping; the other nine are for tents only. An overflow and off-season camping area sits along Flat Fork Creek up from the regular campground. It has only a camping spot and a fire ring. The park gates are closed from sunset to 8 a.m. Late-arriving campers must open and close the gate as they enter. It's best to get situated for the evening and stay within the park's confines. If you plan wisely, you won't even have to get back in your car until you leave for good; there's plenty to do. But if you forgot something, you can purchase supplies back in Wartburg, west on TN 62.

The trails of Frozen Head will take you to some fascinating places. The 3,324-foot Frozen Head Fire Tower is the apex of the trail system. You can see the surrounding highlands of the Cumberland Plateau and the Great Smoky Mountains in the distance. Other features include the Chimney Rock, a natural observation point that looks west as far as the eye can see. Or take the Panther Branch Trail 0.6 miles up to DeBord Falls. A mile farther is Emory Gap Falls. The Lookout Tower and Bird Mountain trails leave directly from the campground. Two miles farther on the Bird Mountain Trail is one of Frozen Head's defining rock formations, Castle Rock. This rock formation is more than 100 feet high and 300 feet wide; with a little imagination you can see the center edifice of the castle with turrets on both ends. These rock formations are the remnants of the erosion-resistant sandstone that covers the Cumberland Plateau. The softer rock and soil below this caprock eroded, leaving rock formations that seemingly jut straight out of the land. Bicyclers can stay on the Lookout Tower Trail and pedal all the way to the fire tower. Hikers can take this trail or one of many others for tower views.

If you don't feel like hiking or relaxing, there are many other activities. Play volleyball on one of the sand courts. Throw horseshoes in one of the three pits. Shoot some basketball at the outdoor court. Check out the free equipment you need at the park office. During the summer, the 240-seat amphitheater hosts many park activities, including interpretive talks, slide shows, movies, and music concerts.

I planned my trip to coincide with spring's wildflower display. Frozen Head has one of the richest

# MAP

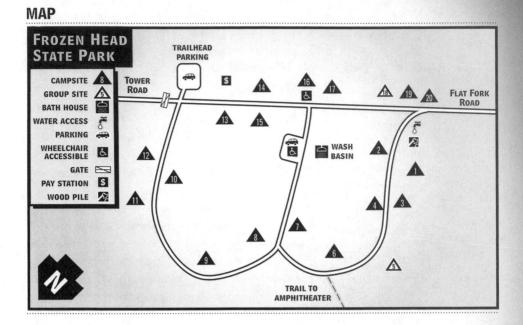

**FROZEN HEAD STATE PARK**

CAMPSITE
GROUP SITE
BATH HOUSE
WATER ACCESS
PARKING
WHEELCHAIR ACCESSIBLE
GATE
PAY STATION
WOOD PILE

TRAILHEAD PARKING

TOWER ROAD

FLAT FORK ROAD

WASH BASIN

TRAIL TO AMPHITHEATER

N

wildflower areas in the Southeast. Even though I could observe purple, yellow, and white symbols of the season directly from my campground, I did tramp many streamside trails and was glad that this piece of the Cumberlands was preserved for all to enjoy.

## GETTING THERE

From Oak Ridge, follow TN 62 west 4 miles to Oliver Springs. Drive 13 miles beyond Oliver Springs and turn right onto Flat Fork Road. A sign for Morgan County Regional Correctional Facility and Frozen Head State Park alerts you to the right turn. Follow Flat Fork Road 4 miles to the entrance of Frozen Head State Park. The visitor center is on your right.

# HIWASSEE-OCOEE
# SCENIC RIVER
# STATE PARK

> *It will take the Hiwassee River and the Gee Creek Wilderness to tear you away from this campground.*

**K**NOWN AS **"GEE CREEK CAMPGROUND,"** the overnighting portion of Hiwassee/Ocoee Scenic River State Park lies in a large, wooded flat at the base of Starr Mountain, adjacent to the cold, clear waters of the Hiwassee River. You can camp out in this high-quality destination and enjoy the Hiwassee River and the trails of the Cherokee National Forest, which abuts the state park. A tall pine forest once shaded the campground but pine beetles decimated them. However, planted hardwoods are growing and providing shade.

The sites are widely spaced along two loops that meander amid the trees. The clean campsites are placed well apart from each other. Even without a lot of groundcover, the sheer number of trees and the distance between sites allow for adequate privacy. You never have to walk too far for water, as spigots are spread out along both loops. The campground is well maintained by state employees. A Tennessee State Park ranger lives opposite the campground.

Gee Creek is open all year, yet it is heavily used only on summer weekends. The bathhouse is located near the center of the campground and is open from mid-March to the end of November. In winter, there are portable toilets, but showers are unavailable; drinking water is provided year-round.

Our visit was during spring. Dogwoods bloomed above the needle-carpeted forest floor. Warm air and cool air played tug-of-war. Squirrels scampered about the campground. Birds flew purposefully from tree to tree. We could sense the rebirth of the mountains around us; it seemed leaves were greening and growing before our very eyes.

The Gee Creek Wilderness is a short distance away and certainly worth a visit. Drive back to US 411 and turn right, then turn right at the sign for Gee

## RATINGS

Beauty: ✿ ✿ ✿ ✿
Privacy: ✿ ✿ ✿ ✿
Spaciousness: ✿ ✿ ✿ ✿ ✿
Quiet: ✿ ✿ ✿
Security: ✿ ✿ ✿ ✿ ✿
Cleanliness: ✿ ✿ ✿ ✿

Creek after half a mile. Follow the paved road over the railroad tracks, then turn right. Drive 2 miles until the road turns to gravel. The Gee Creek Watchable Wildlife Trail is on your left. Just a short distance beyond that is the Gee Creek Trail itself. Trace the old angler's trail up the gorge. Small waterfalls provide plentiful photographic opportunities. The trail crosses the creek several times below old-growth hemlocks and dead-ends after 1.9 miles. On the return trip, look for the little things you missed on the way up. Skilled rock climbers can climb some of the creekside bluffs.

The Gee Creek Watchable Wildlife Trail is a 0.7-mile trail designed to increase the hiker's knowledge of nature's signs. The U.S. Forest Service has placed nest boxes, interpretive information, and wildlife plantings; they have also made a track pit to see which animals have passed by. This is an excellent trail to get children interested in nature. Also starting at the Gee Creek trailhead is the Starr Mountain Trail, number 190. It leads 4.8 miles up to the ridgeline of Starr Mountain and offers expansive views of the surrounding area. The John Muir Trail cruises upstream along the Hiwassee for more than 20 miles, starting just east of the TN 315 bridge over the river near Reliance.

After all this hiking, maybe you need to cool down. Why not enjoy the Hiwassee River? Draining more than 750,000 acres of forested mountain land, it has clear, pure water. Informal trails lead to and along the river from the campground. Make sure young children are supervised. When the turbines upstream are generating, the water will be swift. Most water lovers enjoy the river by raft, canoe, funyak (inflatable kayak), or tube. It's a 5.5-mile float through the splendid Cherokee National Forest. The water, primarily Class I and II on the international scale of difficulty, is very cold. The river is in the last stages of being designated a State Scenic River. Outfitters will supply anything you need, including a shuttle up the river if you have your own equipment. I recommend Hiwassee Outfitters—they are a reputable family operation. Call (800) 338-8133 for information or visit www.hiwasseeoutfitters.com. The nearby Ocoee River has more challenging whitewater.

## KEY INFORMATION

| | |
|---|---|
| ADDRESS: | Box 5 Delano, TN 37325 |
| OPERATED BY: | Tennessee State Parks |
| INFORMATION: | (423) 263-0050; www.tnstateparks.com |
| OPEN: | Year-round |
| SITES: | 43 |
| EACH SITE HAS: | Picnic table, grill, fire pit, lantern post |
| ASSIGNMENT: | First come, first served; no reservations |
| REGISTRATION: | With park staff person on site |
| FACILITIES: | Drinking water, flush toilets, warm showers, soft-drink machines |
| PARKING: | At campsites only |
| FEE: | $12 per night |
| ELEVATION: | 728 feet |
| RESTRICTIONS: | Pets: On leash only Fires: In fire rings only Alcohol: Prohibited Vehicles: None Other: Maximum 14-day stay |

# MAP

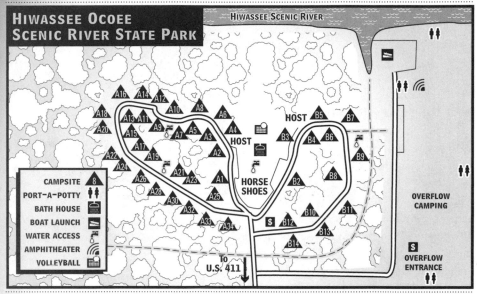

HIWASSEE OCOEE SCENIC RIVER STATE PARK

HIWASSEE SCENIC RIVER

CAMPSITE
PORT-A-POTTY
BATH HOUSE
BOAT LAUNCH
WATER ACCESS
AMPHITHEATER
VOLLEYBALL

HOST

HOST

HORSE SHOES

OVERFLOW CAMPING

OVERFLOW ENTRANCE

To U.S. 411

## GETTING THERE

From Etowah drive 6 miles south on US 411. Turn left onto a signed paved road for Hiwassee/Ocoee Scenic River State Park campground. Pass through an open field with houses. At 1 mile turn right into the campground.

The Hiwassee is also a mecca for those hoping to catch trout. Anglers head to the river on foggy mornings to toss their flies before unsuspecting trout. If you want to try your luck and are ill prepared, there are stores and outfitters nearby who will get you on or in the water. The old train depot town of Etowah is 6 miles north on US 411 if you need supplies.

# HOLLY FLATS

I F YOU PLACE A HIGH PRIORITY on barefoot tent camping, skip Holly Flats. True to its name, the cozy Holly Flats Campground is dotted by holly trees shedding their prickly leaves on the woodland floor. But if you don't mind wearing shoes while you camp, you'll love this place. It offers a variety of sites in a remote place with plenty to do nearby. The Bald River Gorge Wilderness is just across the gravel road, and Waucheesi Mountain and Warriors Passage National Recreation Trail are close as well.

Holly Flats has that old-time campground ambience: the smell of wood smoke and hamburgers cooking; sun filtering through the trees; cool mornings and lazy afternoons. This timeworn feel stems from the simple fact that the campground is old. The picnic tables have their share of initials carved in them, and the fire rings are hand-placed circular piles of rocks. But that's not all bad. The campground is like an old pair of favorite shoes: it may be worn and have a few scuff marks, but it sure is comfortable.

Cross the bridge over Bald River to reach the campground. There are two sites in the grassy area by the bridge for sun lovers. Farther up, the campground splits into two roads that end in small loops. The first road splits off to the right, away from Bald River. It has eight thickly wooded sites spread along a small ridge. These sites offer the most solitude and silence. The farthest site is atop a small hill, away from the road. The second road runs next to Bald River. All six sites are directly riverside in a narrow flat. More open, these campsites lay beneath large trees and have a holly and rhododendron understory. The melody of the river making its descent pervades the flat. A comfort station with vault toilets for each sex is on the side of the road opposite Bald River. Get your water from an old-fashioned hand pump where the two roads split apart.

> *Shoes are a must in this old-time campground next door to the Bald River Wilderness.*

## RATINGS

Beauty: ☆ ☆ ☆ ☆
Privacy: ☆ ☆ ☆ ☆
Spaciousness: ☆ ☆ ☆ ☆ ☆
Quiet: ☆ ☆ ☆ ☆ ☆
Security: ☆ ☆
Cleanliness: ☆ ☆ ☆

| | |
|---|---|
| **ADDRESS:** | 250 Ranger Station Road<br>Tellico Plains, TN 37385 |
| **OPERATED BY:** | Forest Service |
| **INFORMATION:** | (423) 253-2520;<br>www.fs.fed.us/r8/cherokee |
| **OPEN:** | Year-round; access road subject to winter closure |
| **SITES:** | 17 |
| **EACH SITE HAS:** | Tent pad, picnic table, fire ring |
| **ASSIGNMENT:** | First come, first served; no reservations |
| **REGISTRATION:** | Self-registration on site |
| **FACILITIES:** | Hand-pumped water, vault toilet |
| **PARKING:** | At campsites only |
| **FEE:** | $6 per night |
| **ELEVATION:** | 2,150 feet |
| **RESTRICTIONS:** | Pets: On leash only<br>Fires: In fire rings only<br>Alcohol: At campsites only<br>Vehicles: Parking at sites only<br>Other: Pack it in, pack it out |

Holly Flats is a designated pack-it-in, pack-it-out campground. It has no trash receptacles. Pack out all your trash and any trash that thoughtless campers left behind.

Several hiking trails start near Holly Flats. The Bald River Trail (88) starts 0.4 miles west down the Bald River on Forest Service Road 126 and strikes through the heart of the 3,700-acre Bald River Gorge Wilderness. The trail leads 4.8 miles through the steep-sided gorge to Bald River Falls, making for an excellent day hike. For those interested in angling, Bald River is a noted trout stream.

The Kirkland Creek Trail (85) starts 0.4 miles east of the campground on FS 126. A variety of forest types are represented along its route. The trail runs up a valley for 3 miles, then follows an old logging road to Sandy Gap and the North Carolina state line at 4.6 miles.

Less than 1 mile east of Holly Flats on FS 126 is the Brookshire Creek Trail (180). It starts in an old field, crosses Bald River, and climbs 6 miles to the state line. Brookshire Creek has trout as well. Up the trail are some very remote old homesites where, in times past, subsistence mountain farmers cultivated the hills and battled the elements to carve out a living. A clearing lies at the end of the trail and makes a cool summertime picnic spot.

To get a sweat-free overlay of the land, drive to the top of 3,692-foot Waucheesi Mountain. Rangers used to watch for fires from an old tower there. Although the tower has since been torn down, one can still get a view from ground level. From Holly Flats drive west on FS 126 to FS 126C. Turn left and climb the mountain; FS 126C ends at the top. You can peer down into the Bald River Gorge and the Tellico River basin. The Warriors Passage National Recreation Trail (164) starts partway up FS 126C on your right. The trail traces an old route used by the Cherokee on their travels between settlements and, later, by white traders and soldiers who eventually drove the Cherokee out. The historic trail leads to FS 76, 5 miles away. Holly Flats is a relaxing campground bordering one of Tennessee's finest wilderness areas. Give this part of the Cherokee National Forest a look.

## MAP

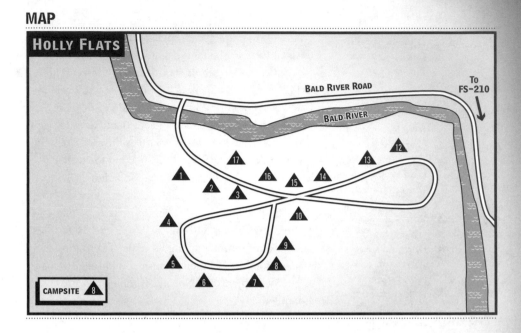

HOLLY FLATS

BALD RIVER ROAD

To FS-210

BALD RIVER

CAMPSITE 8

## GETTING THERE

From Tellico Plains drive
5.3 miles east on TN 165.
Turn right onto FS 210 and
go 13.9 miles to FS 126. Turn
right onto the gravel FS 126
and follow it 6 miles. Holly
Flats Campground will be
across a bridge on your left.

# INDIAN BOUNDARY

> *Indian Boundary is the pride of the Cherokee National Forest.*

**I**NDIAN **B**OUNDARY **IS THE PRIDE** of the southern Cherokee National Forest. And with good reason— the wooded camping area lies in a flat beside a clear lake and is overlooked by mountains. Individual campsites are tastefully integrated into the natural beauty of the land adjacent to Flats Mountain. Nearby recreational opportunities center around, but are not limited to, Indian Boundary Lake. Some developments, including warm showers throughout the campground and electricity in one loop, make for a less-rustic atmosphere, but this campground can be a great choice for seasoned tent campers who want to bring their more citified friends and relatives.

The main campground is divided into four loops. Loop A is closest to Indian Boundary Lake. A pine-and-oak forest cloaks the rolling hills here, making for a good combination of sun and shade. As with all the loops, a campground host is there to help campers enjoy their stay. Two comfort stations here have warm showers.

Loop B is the domain of the RVers. Why? In a word, electricity. This is one of two electrified loops, so the big rigs congregate here as well as in Loop C, which is also electric. Gravel is spread between the leveled sites and landscaping timbers. Overhead are tall white pines and oaks. Tent campers have better options on Loops A and D. Loop C and Loop D interconnect beneath rolling pine woods bisected by a small creek bed, but they are farthest from the lake, which is the focus of recreation here. The Overflow Loop, open year-round, is more spacious, with a grassy central area surrounded by woods.

Anglers enjoy bank fishing or launching a boat into the clear waters here. The atmosphere stays quiet because no gas motors are allowed. The view of the surrounding mountains from the lake may distract

## RATINGS

Beauty: ✿ ✿ ✿ ✿ ✿
Privacy: ✿ ✿ ✿
Spaciousness: ✿ ✿ ✿
Quiet: ✿ ✿ ✿ ✿
Security: ✿ ✿ ✿ ✿
Cleanliness: ✿ ✿ ✿ ✿

anglers from vying for largemouth bass, trout, and bream or the tackle-busting catfish that purportedly wait down deep. There is a swimming beach along one section of the impoundment. The Lakeshore Trail makes a 3.2-mile loop around Indian Boundary Lake.

More ambitious hikers have the Citico Creek Wilderness in which to tramp. Just a piece down Forest Service Road 35-1 is the South Fork Citico Creek trailhead. Here, hikers can make loops involving the Brush Mountain, Pine Ridge, and North and South Fork Citico Creek trails. Stream anglers can enjoy the wild setting while casting a line for native trout in Citico Creek and its tributaries. A helpful map of the Citico Creek Wilderness is available at the nearby Tellico Ranger Station.

Campers reach Indian Boundary via the Cherohala Skyway. This scenic road rivals the Blue Ridge Parkway or Newfound Gap Road in the Smokies for scenery. Uphill from Indian Boundary, scenic overlooks dot the way to Beech Gap and beyond the North Carolina state line. Also at Beech Gap is the Fodderstack Trail. This path traces an old road for a distance then climbs up to Bob Bald, a mile-high open meadow. An easier hike is the one to Hooper Bald; the trail lies a little farther along the Cherohala Skyway. Take a short nature trail to reach this meadow at 5,300 feet. More views await at nearby Huckleberry Knob. An informative handout on the skyway is also available at the Tellico Ranger Station.

Indian Boundary is a popular destination. Expect a full campground during the peak summer season. A reservation system can guarantee you a campsite up to 240 days in advance. There are less crowded times to visit, though. Consider coming here in May. Fall is also a good choice; leaf viewers are likely to see vibrant colors, since the Cherohala Skyway traverses elevations from less than 1,000 feet to more than 5,000 feet. No matter what time of year, you should head for the borders of Indian Boundary.

## KEY INFORMATION

| | |
|---|---|
| **ADDRESS:** | 250 Ranger Station Road, Tellico Plains, TN 37385 |
| **OPERATED BY:** | Forest Service |
| **INFORMATION:** | (423) 253-2520; www.fs.fed.us/r8/cherokee |
| **OPEN:** | Main campground, mid-April– October; overflow area, year-round |
| **SITES:** | 95 |
| **EACH SITE HAS:** | Picnic table, fire grate, lantern post, electricity on Loops B and C |
| **ASSIGNMENT:** | Some sites by reservation; others are first come, first served |
| **REGISTRATION:** | By phone or on site; reserve by phone (877) 444-6777 or online www.reserve usa.com |
| **FACILITIES:** | Water spigot, warm showers, flush toilet |
| **PARKING:** | At campsites only |
| **FEE:** | $20 per night |
| **ELEVATION:** | 1,800 feet |
| **RESTRICTIONS:** | Pets: On leash only; Fires: In fire grates only; Alcohol: At campsites only; Vehicles: Maximum 25-foot-long trailers; Other: Maximum 14-day stay |

## MAP

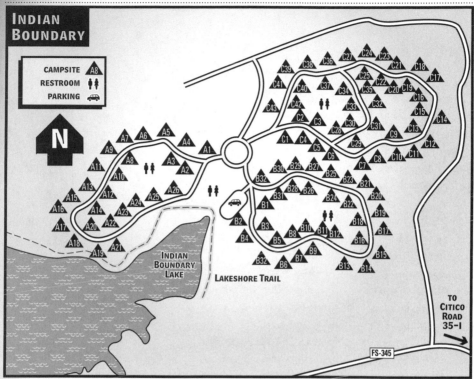

INDIAN BOUNDARY

CAMPSITE A8
RESTROOM 👫
PARKING 🚗

N

INDIAN BOUNDARY LAKE
LAKESHORE TRAIL

TO CITICO ROAD 35-I

FS-345

## GETTING THERE

From the town square in Tellico Plains, drive south on TN 165, known as Cherohala Skyway, 14 miles to Forest Service Road 345. Turn left onto FS 345 and follow it 1 mile into the Indian Boundary Recreation Area.

# JAKE BEST

**JAKE BEST CAMPGROUND LIES** in wooded solitude on a bluff overlooking Citico Creek. The seven sites are spaciously arranged along a gravel loop road. The two most popular sites are creekside, below the bluff. Though the isolated encampment lies in hilly terrain, the sites are level and well separated from one another. With so few sites, you'll never be bothered by the endless drone of other car campers coming and going along the loop road.

> *Jake Best makes a peaceful headquarters for exploring nearby Citico Creek Wilderness.*

The campground and nearby stream are named for Jake Best, a settler from the mid-1800s; his house up the creek bears his name. A clearing and some graves still mark the homesite. The camping area is fairly open by Southern Appalachian standards, but some trees were left to provide ample shade and privacy. The allure of Jake Best is its primitive setting. You're one with nature here. In fact, a "bear country" notice is posted at the fee area, so do not let too much distance get between you and your food. Because the pump well has been disconnected, you will need to get your water from the creek; be sure to treat or boil all water before consuming it. During my Jake Best experience, I got up one morning and stumbled down to the creek to get water for coffee. In my sleepy state I actually stumbled into the creek, soaking my lower half. That did a better job of waking me up than the coffee would have!

Only 10 miles as the crow flies from the Great Smoky Mountains National Park, this rustic campground offers visitors scenery and history that rival that of the national park itself. In years past, this was Cherokee country, so many area landmarks bear native Indian names. The name Citico is derived from the Cherokee word *sitiku,* which means "clean fishing waters." The name's claim holds. The clear water of Citico Creek has quite a nip to it, even in summer.

## RATINGS

Beauty: ✩ ✩ ✩ ✩
Privacy: ✩ ✩ ✩
Spaciousness: ✩ ✩ ✩ ✩ ✩
Quiet: ✩ ✩ ✩ ✩ ✩
Security: ✩ ✩ ✩ ✩
Cleanliness: ✩ ✩ ✩

## KEY INFORMATION

**ADDRESS:** 250 Ranger Station Road
Tellico Plains, TN 37385

**OPERATED BY:** Forest Service

**INFORMATION:** (423) 253-2520; www.fs.fed.us/r8/cherokee

**OPEN:** Year-round

**SITES:** 7

**EACH SITE HAS:** Graveled tent pad, picnic table, rock fire ring, lantern post, trash can

**ASSIGNMENT:** First come, first served; no reservations

**REGISTRATION:** Self-registration on site

**FACILITIES:** Pit toilet

**PARKING:** At individual sites

**FEE:** $6 per night

**ELEVATION:** 1,300 feet

**RESTRICTIONS:** Pets: On leash or under physical control
Fires: In fire rings only
Alcohol: At campsites only
Vehicles: At campsites only
Other: Maximum 14-day stay

After the Cherokee came the lumberjack. The logging era lasted into the 1920s. A railroad ran along Citico Creek and its tributaries; its remains can still be seen today. The logging harvest devastated the land through a series of clear-cuts, stream siltings, and wildfires. When the logging stopped, settlers moved in. Then the Forest Service bought the land. A Civilian Conservation Corps camp was converted into the campground we see today. The surrounding watershed is returning to its former natural character—so much so that in 1984 the upper section of the Citico Creek watershed was recognized for its exceptional beauty and was designated a wilderness.

Jake Best Campground is an ideal base camp for exploring the Citico Wilderness. A map of the southern half of the Cherokee National Forest comes in very handy. A series of trails leave from Doublecamp Road, Forest Service Road 59. From Jake Best drive 4 miles up Citico Creek Road (FS 35-1). Turn left to reach FS 59. Having hiked and camped throughout this wilderness, I strongly recommend the following hikes.

The Crowder Branch Trail (84) starts 3.5 miles up FS 59. It leads 2.6 miles along a charming mountain stream through impressive woods to end at Crowder Place. An old homesite, Crowder Place has a reliable spring and an open meadow for your picnicking pleasure. At 6.7 miles on FS 59 you'll find Farr Gap and the Fodderstack Trail. The path leads along Fodderstack Ridge, affording intermittent views of the surrounding wilderness and the Smokies beyond.

Drive 5.6 miles up Citico Creek Road, FS 35-1, then go left a short distance on FS 26 to the jumping off point for numerous trailheads that lead into the wilderness. Take the South Fork Citico Trail (105) and delve deep into the mountains. The old, square building with no roof was once the camp commissary and powder magazine for the logging camp known as Jeffrey. Other history, both human and natural, awaits you down the trail.

On our trip here, during a late-winter weekend, we had the campground to ourselves. We chose a sunny site, enjoying those first warm rays that signal the impending arrival of spring. That night, a full

## MAP

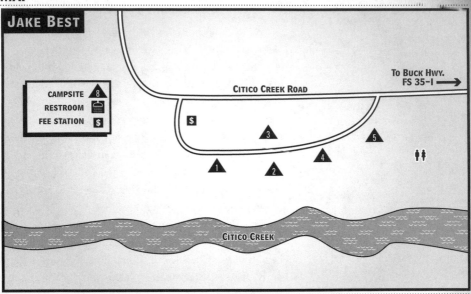

JAKE BEST

CAMPSITE ▲ 8
RESTROOM 🚻
FEE STATION 💲

CITICO CREEK ROAD

To Buck Hwy.
FS 35-1 →

💲

▲ 3

▲ 5

▲ 4

▲ 1

▲ 2

🚻

CITICO CREEK

moon rose over Cowcamp Ridge and shone so brightly we cooked our supper over the fire without any artificial light.

Try to bring in all your supplies, as Jake Best is pretty far from the civilized world. And that can be good. You will enjoy this land that probably would have been a national park itself had the unmatched Smokies not been so close.

## GETTING THERE

From the town square in Tellico Plains, drive 0.5 miles south on TN 165. Turn left onto TN 360 and drive 9 miles to Monroe County 504, also known as Buck Highway. Make a right at the sign to Citico Creek, then drive 5.1 miles to FS 35-1. Along the way, make sure to veer left at the junction with Monroe County 506. After turning right on FS 35-1, drive 2.9 miles to Jake Best Campground on your left.

# LITTLE OAK

> *Picking the best of these sites will be your biggest problem at Little Oak.*

**L**AKESIDE CAMPING IS A BREEZE at Little Oak. The camp is sizable and well laid out, situated atop what was left of Little Oak Mountain after the Holston River Valley was flooded to create South Holston Lake. Though large, Little Oak is widely dispersed on four loops that jut into the lake. This arrangement allows for many spacious lakeside sites, and each loop feels like its own little campground. Short paths slope from each lakeside site to the water's edge. There are many attractive sites from which to choose. We drove each loop so many times, seeing one ideal site and then seeing an even better one, that we were sure another camper was going to turn our license plate in to a ranger. This campground was designed for a pleasant camping experience, not just as a way station for the urban masses.

Just beyond the pay station is Hemlock Loop, which contains 14 sites nestled beneath a thick stand of hemlock trees. Most of the sites are on the outside of the loop, well away from one another, with plenty of cover between sites. An old-fashioned vault toilet and a modern comfort station with flush toilets and showers are at the head of the loop. Camp at Hemlock Loop if you like very shady sites.

Lone Pine Loop is for those who prefer sunny sites. There are two small fields adjacent to the loop that allow more light into the camping areas. Three comfort stations are located by the 16 sites. Only the northern end of the loop has lakeside sites.

Big Oak Loop has 16 sites and is located on a spit of hardwoods and evergreens that juts north into the lake. Nearly all the sites are lakeside. A modern comfort station is located halfway along the loop, and water faucets are nearby. The view from Big Oak Loop into South Holston Lake is my personal favorite.

Poplar Loop is the largest loop, with 23 sites, but

## RATINGS

Beauty: ✪ ✪ ✪ ✪
Privacy: ✪ ✪ ✪ ✪
Spaciousness: ✪ ✪ ✪ ✪ ✪
Quiet: ✪ ✪ ✪
Security: ✪ ✪ ✪ ✪ ✪
Cleanliness: ✪ ✪ ✪ ✪

the sites are split into two loops of their own, facing west and south into the lake. There is a modern comfort station at each loop. Most of these sites are lakeside.

We finally settled on Big Oak Loop. After setting up camp, we watched the sun turn into a red ball of fire over South Holston Lake. Gentle waves lapped at our feet as we sat on the shoreline. We took a vigorous hike in the cool of the next morning on the Little Oak Trail that loops the outer peninsula of the campground. This campground is virtually surrounded by the lake, which gives it an aquatic ambience. For a different perspective, take the Little Oak Mountain Trail. It leaves the campground near the pay station and circles back after dipping into the woods. For yet another perspective on Little Oak, get out on the lake itself. A boat ramp is conveniently situated between the Hemlock and Poplar loops. Swim, fish, or take a pleasure ride up the lake into Virginia.

In East Tennessee, the high country is never far away. Little Oak is near the Flint Mill Scenic Area, which has a broad representation of Southern Appalachian flora and fauna and elevations exceeding 4,000 feet. Turn right out of the campground onto Forest Service Road 87 and drive a short 1.4 miles. The Josiah Trail (Forest Trail 50) starts on your left and ascends 2.2 miles to a saddle on Holston Mountain and Forest Trail 44. To your right after 3.4 miles is the Holston Mountain Fire Tower and views aplenty. Flint Mill Trail (Forest Trail 49) climbs one steep mile to Flint Rock and some fantastic views of South Holston Lake. The trail is 2.2 miles on the left beyond the Josiah Trail. Fishing equipment and other supplies are available back in Bristol.

## KEY INFORMATION

| | |
|---|---|
| ADDRESS: | 4400 Unicoi Drive Unicoi, TN 37692 |
| OPERATED BY: | Forest Service |
| INFORMATION: | (423) 735-1500; www.fs.fed.us/r8/cherokee |
| OPEN: | Late April–November |
| SITES: | 72 |
| EACH SITE HAS: | Tent pad, picnic table, fire ring, lantern post |
| ASSIGNMENT: | First come, first served; no reservations |
| REGISTRATION: | Self-registration on site |
| FACILITIES: | Water faucets, flush toilets, warm showers |
| PARKING: | At campsites only |
| FEE: | $12 per night; $6 when running water is unavailable |
| ELEVATION: | 1,750 feet |
| RESTRICTIONS: | Pets: On leash only Fires: In fire rings only Alcohol: Prohibited Vehicles: None Other: Maximum 14-day stay |

## MAP

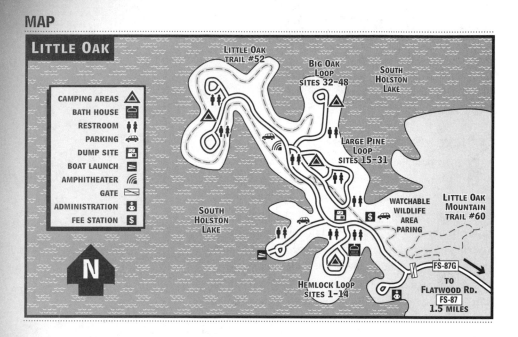

**LITTLE OAK**

LITTLE OAK
TRAIL #52

BIG OAK
LOOP
SITES 32-48

SOUTH
HOLSTON
LAKE

CAMPING AREAS
BATH HOUSE
RESTROOM
PARKING
DUMP SITE
BOAT LAUNCH
AMPHITHEATER
GATE
ADMINISTRATION
FEE STATION

LARGE PINE
LOOP
SITES 15-31

SOUTH
HOLSTON
LAKE

WATCHABLE
WILDLIFE
AREA
PARING

LITTLE OAK
MOUNTAIN
TRAIL #60

N

HEMLOCK LOOP
SITES 1-14

FS-87G

TO
FLATWOOD RD.
FS-87
1.5 MILES

## GETTING THERE

From Bristol, take US 421 east 14 miles. Turn right onto Camp Tom Howard Road (FS 87) at the signed intersection for Little Oak Campground. Follow FS 87 about 6.5 miles. Turn right onto FS 87G and follow it 1.5 miles to dead-end into Little Oak Recreation Area.

# NOLICHUCKY GORGE

**T**HE **NOLICHUCKY RIVER CUTS** a deep gorge through the Appalachian Mountains as it flows from North Carolina into Tennessee. Frothing whitewater tumbles over rocks and boulders beneath towering green ridges. Just a short distance into the Volunteer State, Jones Branch flows into the Nolichucky, creating a riverside flat where Rick Murray, rafter and whitewater man extraordinaire, located his Nolichucky Gorge Campground. This flat, overlooking the river, is surrounded by national forest land, with the exception of a rafting company located next door. Having such a neighbor enhances the camping experience here, as rafting the Nolichucky is the primary recreational activity in the gorge. Furthermore, the long-distance Appalachian Trail passes a mere 50 yards from your campsite, offering hiking opportunities. Don't feel like pitching your own tent? Rick has installed platform tents—cabin-style tents elevated above the ground on wooden platforms and equipped with air mattresses to make your camp out even more convenient. One more thing: the fishing here can be very good.

Let us start with the campground. Cross Jones Branch on a small bridge and enter the camping area. Along both sides of the creek are shaded campsites equipped with platform tents. To the right is the river. Nine campsites that offer ideal access and even better views of the mountains beyond are stretched along the water. Some sites are shaded; others are more in the open. A grassy lawn provides the understory. To your left is a gravel loop road. Here is the campground office, eight RV sites, and four tent sites that are mostly in the open. Backing up to the hillside are five shaded tent sites. Also back here are nine platform tent sites deep in the shade of pine and tulip trees. Deep in more pines are a dozen more tent sites that shade lovers will snap up. An open understory diminishes

> *Raft, hike, fish, and camp in the deep gorge of the Nolichucky River.*

## RATINGS

Beauty: ✮ ✮ ✮ ✮
Privacy: ✮ ✮ ✮
Spaciousness: ✮ ✮ ✮ ✮
Quiet: ✮ ✮ ✮ ✮
Security: ✮ ✮ ✮ ✮
Cleanliness: ✮ ✮ ✮ ✮ ✮

## KEY INFORMATION

campsite privacy. Most sites rate above average on spaciousness. The bathhouse is located near the campground office. Nolichucky Gorge encourages reservations, and I do too. When the water is high the campground can fill because the Nolichucky Gorge is all about whitewater.

The primary rafting run starts in North Carolina, 9 miles upstream. This run offers Class III and IV whitewater and gorge-ous scenery. The "Noli," as it is known among whitewater aficionados, streams from the slopes of Mount Mitchell, the highest point in the East, and slices through the Unaka Mountains. The Unakas are mostly forested, with serrated outcrops of stone jutting above the wood. Being on national forest land gives the river run a wild and natural aura. Many folks bring their own kayaks and whitewater canoes. Increasing in popularity these days are "funyaks," inflatable kayaks. If you don't have your own boat, walk across Jones Branch to USA Raft. This rafting company uses self-bailing rafts that drain the water as it splashes overboard. You can also tube downstream from the campground in milder water that is primarily Class II in difficulty.

You can enjoy the water without a boat as well. Take a trail from the campground heading upstream along the river to the campground swimming beach. This way you can intentionally take a dip instead of taking one falling overboard. You can also fish the Nolichucky. Trout swim the refreshing waters, as do smallmouth bass, catfish, and muskellunge. Land-based recreation focuses on the Appalachian Trail. Southbound hikers can wind their way along the steep cliffs of the Nolichucky Gorge 1.3 miles to reach the bridge crossing the river over which you drove to get to the campground. It's a steep climb if you keep going, but you will be rewarded with fine views of the Nolichucky Gorge. Northbound hikers will ascend from the river to eventually reach Curley Maple Gap trail shelter after 3 miles and Indian Grave Gap 4 miles beyond that. Unless you have a backpack and sleeping bag you will have a hard time making it all the way to Maine. So head on back to the Nolichucky Gorge, a fine place to be, whether you are hiking, fishing, or rafting.

## MAP

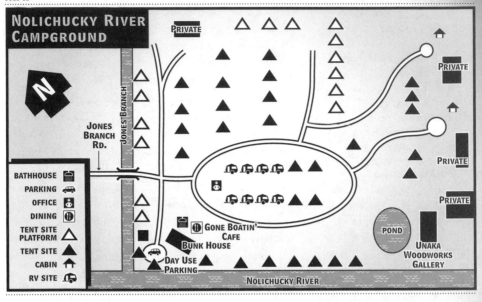

**NOLICHUCKY RIVER CAMPGROUND**

PRIVATE

JONES BRANCH RD.

JONES BRANCH

BATHHOUSE
PARKING
OFFICE
DINING
TENT SITE PLATFORM
TENT SITE
CABIN
RV SITE

PRIVATE

PRIVATE

PRIVATE

PRIVATE

POND

UNAKA WOODWORKS GALLERY

GONE BOATIN' CAFE
BUNK HOUSE

DAY USE PARKING

NOLICHUCKY RIVER

## GETTING THERE

From Exit 15 on I-26 near Erwin, head east on Jackson–Love Highway just a short distance to Temple Hill Road. Turn right on Temple Hill Road and follow it 0.5 miles to River Road. Turn left on River Road and follow it 0.5 miles to Chestoa Pike. Turn left on Chestoa Pike and cross the Nolichucky River to reach Jones Branch Road, immediately on your right. Turn right onto Jones Branch Road and follow it 1.3 miles to dead-end at the campground, just beyond the rafting center.

# NORRIS DAM
# STATE PARK

> *Relics of pioneer history and outdoor recreational activities abound around the site of the Tennessee Valley Authority's first dam.*

**T**HERE IS SO MUCH TO DO at Norris Dam State Park and environs that it's hard to know where to begin. What started as a flood-control project in the Great Depression has resulted in a park with a lake, a river, and land recreation administered by the State of Tennessee and the Tennessee Valley Authority, more commonly referred to as the TVA. During the flood-control project's development, the pioneer history of the Clinch River Valley was evident, thus a special emphasis was placed on preserving the past as changes were made. Today, we have the Lenoir Pioneer Museum, an 18th-century gristmill, a threshing barn, and, outside the park boundaries, one of East Tennessee's most rewarding attractions, the Museum of Appalachia.

But there is a drawback. The two park campgrounds are only just above run-of-the mill. In fact, it isn't worth looking for a site at West Campground, at least for us tent campers. However, the East Campground has a primitive area that makes the overnighting experience here better than tolerable. Coming from Norris, you will turn right into the eastern park entrance just before reaching the dam. Drive on up and turn into the East Campground. It is a little too cramped and open, and it is under a power line. Not good. Paved pads, water, and electricity make this RV heaven. But some sites are adequately spaced, and a determined tent camper can find a place to camp here. A road spurs right, down to thick woods. This is the Primitive Camping Area. Here in the shade are informal sites, not numbered, with picnic tables and rock fire rings. Most of the sites are level enough to let you avoid tossing and turning at night. There are additional sites adjacent to the gravel loop road that climbs back toward the main campground. A campsite atop the hill by the power line is appealing for its solitude. There is

## RATINGS

Beauty: ✪ ✪
Privacy: ✪ ✪ ✪
Spaciousness: ✪ ✪ ✪ ✪
Quiet: ✪ ✪ ✪ ✪
Security: ✪ ✪ ✪ ✪
Cleanliness: ✪ ✪ ✪ ✪

a bathhouse in the center of the main camping loop. Primitive sites are available year-round, except on holiday weekends. The West Campground is a few miles distant. It has 50 overly crowded RV sites atop a hill that has too little shade. Don't bother unless you are sizing up RVs to buy.

Now to the good stuff. Norris Lake, the result of Norris Dam, is one of the most attractive lakes in the South. A boating experience of any kind is bound to be a good one, whether it is for skiing, fishing, or just pleasure cruising. A commercial marina, on the far side of the dam from East Campground, will serve your boating needs. The Clinch River flows from beneath the dam. Many die-hard anglers tout its cold waters as the finest trout fishing in the state. I have enjoyed many float-fishing trips down this river and have caught my share of trout.

If you are more land-oriented, paths galore will keep you coming back for more. Four distinct trail systems course through the area. The Civilian Conservation Corps Camp Trail System, developed in the 1930s along with the dam, is near the East Campground. Several interconnected trails mean a number of loops are possible. The High Point Trail extends nearly 4 miles and is open to mountain bikes. The Andrews Ridge Trail System is near the West Campground. It winds through a younger forest that was once the farmland of families relocated during the damming. The Park Headquarters Trail System has a fitness trail with exercise stations. The TVA Trail System includes the River Bluff Trail, which travels along the Clinch River.

History buffs should visit the privately owned Museum of Appalachia. The owner, John Rice Irwin, truly takes pride in this region, and it shows at this 65-acre destination that must be seen to be appreciated. Inside Norris Dam State Park's boundaries is the Lenoir Museum. It gives a pictorial history of the area in pre-dam days. Nearby are the threshing barn and an old gristmill, which operates during the summer. Ranger-led activities, conducted Wednesday through Sunday in summer, include rappelling, making trips to Hill Cave, and cruising the lake to learn more about the history of Norris Dam. One thing you won't hear

## KEY INFORMATION

**ADDRESS:** 125 Village Green Circle
Lake City, TN 37769

**OPERATED BY:** Tennessee State Parks

**INFORMATION:** (865) 426-7461; www.tnstateparks.com

**OPEN:** Year-round

**SITES:** East Campground 10 primitive, 25 nonprimitive; West Campground 50 nonprimitive

**EACH SITE HAS:** Picnic table, fire ring (primitive sites); water and electricity (nonprimitive sites)

**ASSIGNMENT:** First come, first served; no reservations

**REGISTRATION:** At park office, or ranger will come by to register you

**FACILITIES:** Hot showers, flush toilets, water spigots, laundry, pay phone

**PARKING:** At campsites only

**FEE:** Tents, $17.50 April–October, $15.50 November–March

**ELEVATION:** 1,100 feet

**RESTRICTIONS:** Pets: On 6-foot leash only
Fires: In fire rings only
Alcohol: Prohibited
Vehicles: Bikes, minibikes, and ATVs prohibited
Other: Maximum 14-day stay

## MAP

NORRIS DAM STATE PARK

**N**

CAMPSITE — 8
BATH HOUSE
RANGER RESIDENCE
TELEPHONE
PLAYGROUND

PRIMITIVE SITES

A · C · B

ANDREWS RIDGE TRAIL

HOOTIN HOLLOW TRAIL

TO 441

EAST CAMPING AREA

WEST CAMPING AREA

NON-CONTIGUOUS

TO 441

CAMPER CHECK-IN

**N**

## GETTING THERE

From Exit 122 on I-75 near Norris, head 1.4 miles west on TN 61 to US 441. Turn left on 441 and follow it 6 miles to East Campground adjacent to Norris Dam.

on a tent-camping trip here is, "I'm bored. There's nothing to do."

# NORTH RIVER

**N**ORTH RIVER CAMPGROUND is located deep within the Cherokee National Forest. The campground, situated on a level river bend between a wooded mountainside and the clear-running North River, has a serene atmosphere. For a tent camper who likes minimum fanfare and maximum nature, this is the place. Human accoutrements are sparse in this Forest Service camping area, but natural amenities are abundant. Trout swim the creek's waters shaded by hemlock, sycamore, and rhododendron. Mature dogwoods and white pine provide a beautiful backdrop for those relaxing evenings fireside. There are grassy areas between the trees, accentuating the ample spaciousness between the level tent sites. Dead, fallen firewood is abundant in the area, as are nature's citizens: deer, wild turkey, wild boar, and bear.

With only 11 sites in the entire campground, quiet rules here. The North River will lull you to sleep at night and the birds will be your alarm clock in the morning. For the water lover, 8 of the 11 sites are riverside. Two of the sites could qualify as group sites, with double picnic tables, additional tent pads, and ample parking for families. In contrast, the lower end of the campground is shadier and more isolated, while the upper end is sunnier and more open. Bathroom facilities are spartan, with one pit toilet for each sex. An old-fashioned hand-pump well sits in the middle of the campground. Pump the green handle to fill your pots and pans. If the amenities sound too coarse, remember that this is a place to come to relish the out-of-doors and a past way of life.

Beard cane, a species of grass, grows alongside the North River in the campground. The leaves on the main stem of the cane form the plant's "beard." Mountaineers once used the plant for fishing poles. Modern-day anglers prefer to fly-fish and are inspired by a trip

> *Let this slice of river in Southern Appalachia be your quiet woodland escape.*

## RATINGS

Beauty: ☆ ☆ ☆ ☆ ☆
Privacy: ☆ ☆ ☆ ☆
Spaciousness: ☆ ☆ ☆ ☆ ☆
Quiet: ☆ ☆ ☆ ☆
Security: ☆ ☆ ☆
Cleanliness: ☆ ☆ ☆

**ADDRESS:** 250 Ranger Station Road
Tellico Plains, TN 37385

**OPERATED BY:** Forest Service

**INFORMATION:** (423) 253-2520; www.fs.fed.us/r8/cherokee

**OPEN:** Year-round

**SITES:** 11

**EACH SITE HAS:** Graveled tent pad, picnic table, fire ring, lantern holder

**ASSIGNMENT:** First come, first served; no reservations

**REGISTRATION:** Self-registration on site

**FACILITIES:** Hand-pumped water, pit toilet

**PARKING:** At individual sites

**FEE:** $8 per night

**ELEVATION:** 1,840 feet

**RESTRICTIONS:** Pets: On leash or under physical control
Fires: In fire rings only
Alcohol: At campsites only
Vehicles: At campsites only
Other: Maximum 14-day stay

to the nearby Pheasant Fields Fish Hatchery, 4.5 miles away. Turn right out of the campground and turn right again 0.1 mile down Forest Service Road 216. Go 1 mile and turn left up FS 210, then travel 3.5 miles. Rainbow trout are raised at the hatchery for stocking, and in one of the many tanks there are some lunkers that will cause your eyes to pop in disbelief. If you get the urge to explore, stretch your legs on the Sycamore Creek Trail (Forest Trail 61), which starts at the fish hatchery. Sycamore Creek is the feeder stream for the hatchery. The trail leads up to Whigg Meadow, an open field nearly a mile high, sporting views into Citico Creek and Slickrock Wilderness. Nearby, down FS 217 from the campground, are the McNabb and Hemlock Creek trails (92 and 101, respectively). These trails are located in the Brushy Ridge Primitive Area just across from the campground. Each footpath follows a scenic tributary of the North River up to the high country. Before darkness falls, grab your camera and drive back to Bald River Falls for some scenic shots of this panoramic waterfall.

While exploring the area, my friends and I came to a rough road a few miles beyond the hatchery, just over the North Carolina line. We followed it for a distance because I wanted to show them where I had become stuck fording the Tellico River. As we came upon the crossing, we found a frustrated couple standing by their four-wheel-drive vehicle: It was stuck in the very place that mine had been stuck a decade earlier! We pulled them out with a chain and turned around, laughing at the irony of the situation.

During the summer you can purchase supplies in the small community of Green Cove. It is an inholding in the national forest, consisting of summer cottages, a little motel, a small country store, and a gas station. Green Cove is located two miles from the campground up FS 210 before the fish hatchery.

If you want to camp in a national forest surrounded by natural beauty, come to the North River Campground. Literally encircled by mountainous woodland, it is spacious enough that you never feel packed in. Fellow campers are likely to be friendly locals from Monroe County who will help you in any way they can.

## MAP

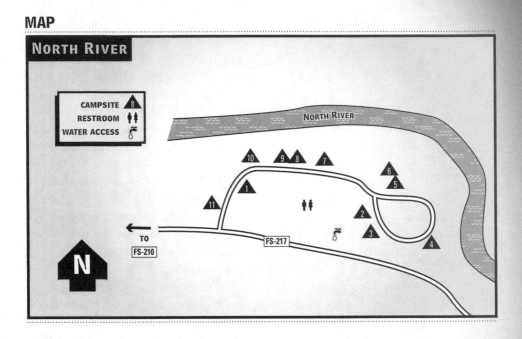

NORTH RIVER

CAMPSITE 8
RESTROOM
WATER ACCESS

NORTH RIVER

10   9  8      7
          6
           5
    1
11
            2
          3
               4
TO
FS-210        FS-217

N

## GETTING THERE

From the town square in Tellico Plains, drive 4.7 miles south on TN 165 to FS 210. Turn right onto FS 210 and drive 9.6 miles to FS 217, passing Tellico Ranger Station at 0.4 miles, where you might want to obtain a forest map. Also pass Bald River Falls at 6.3 miles. Turn left 3.3 miles past the falls on FS 217. Follow FS 217 about 3 miles. North River Campground will be on your right.

# OBED WILD AND SCENIC RIVER

*Enjoy the wonders of the wild and scenic Obed River from this new campground.*

THE OBED NATIONAL WILD AND SCENIC River, administered by the National Park Service, has come of age. What was once a protected recreation area in name only has now evolved into a multiple-outdoor-activity destination supported by the community. It all began with die-hard kayakers and canoers plying the whitewater of the Obed–Emory River watershed. Next a few paddle access points were established. Then a 14-mile segment of the Cumberland Trail, which runs through the heart of the Obed River gorge, was completed. The addition of Rock Creek Campground at the Nemo Bridge boat access has made this scenic swath of the Cumberland Plateau a prime destination for tent campers.

When I started coming here nearly two decades ago, the Nemo Bridge area was a local party spot. Boy, have things changed. The old boat access is now a nice picnic area and trailhead. The old Nemo Bridge is used for foot traffic only. Continue across the new bridge, turn right, and descend into the campground after crossing clear Rock Creek. Dead ahead is the self-service fee station. To the left is a single campsite that offers the most privacy. Enter a tall woodland of sycamore and tulip trees, and pass the Cumberland Trail, which conveniently leaves directly from the camping area. One site lies near the trail. Pass two vault toilets, and then come to two nice campsites that are just a stone's throw from the Obed River. A nature trail heads upriver beyond these two campsites.

The high-quality design of Rock Creek Campground is immediately evident, with the landscaping timbers delineating the sites, which have raised tent pads of coarse sand that offer quick drainage and easy staking. The stone picnic tables are embellished with designs, much as you would see in a garden at home. The fire rings and lantern posts are placed to last a

## RATINGS

Beauty: ✿ ✿ ✿ ✿ ✿
Privacy: ✿ ✿ ✿
Spaciousness: ✿ ✿ ✿
Quiet: ✿ ✿ ✿ ✿
Security: ✿ ✿ ✿
Cleanliness: ✿ ✿ ✿ ✿

long time. Curve along the river and come to campsite 5. It is also close to the river and near Rock Creek as well. Pass two more good sites then come to a set of three walk-in tent campsites. Two wooden bridges span a wet-weather drainage to access the shady sites that feature some hemlocks and rhododendron. The final site is handicap-accessible. Campers should be able to find a site most any weekend if they arrive on Friday. Getting a site is no problem during the week and in the fall and winter. Summer weekdays are good, too. Plan to scramble for a site on spring weekends when the water is right for paddling.

So what about all the great recreation here? The Obed is really comprised of four drainages that offer paddling of all difficulties. These watercourses— Daddy's Creek, Clear Creek, Emory River, and the Obed River—have cut gorges into the Cumberland Plateau, where bluffs overlook rock-choked rivers running through thick forests. Upper Daddy's Creek is for experts only, but the last 2 miles, from the Devils Breakfast Table onward are Class II water, as is the Emory River from Nemo Bridge to Oakdale, which leaves takes one across the park's boundary. Just watch for that first rapid, Nemo: it has flipped me a few times. Some sections of Clear Creek are doable by average boaters, but other runs are tough. If you are going to paddle, on your initial trips go with someone who knows the water, and call the visitor center for water levels.

The rivers are good for fishing, too. Muskie, bass, bream and catfish, await in the river's deeper holes; most of these are accessible by self-propelled boat or foot only. This National Park Service destination also has a good walk for you: Take the Cumberland Trail from the campground up the Emory River, climbing away from the water before it reaches its confluence with the Obed. At 2.6 miles you will near Alley Ford. Another 2 miles will take you to Breakaway Bluff Overlook. The trail travels on to Rock Garden Overlook and views of rapids before picking up an old railroad bed. The 14-mile trail ends at the Devils Breakfast Table on Daddy's Creek. If this one-way trek is too far, consider driving to the Devils Breakfast Table and

## KEY INFORMATION

| | |
|---|---|
| **ADDRESS:** | P.O. Box 429, 208 North Maiden Street Wartburg, TN 37887 |
| **OPERATED BY:** | National Park Service |
| **INFORMATION:** | (423) 346-6294; www.nps.gov/obed |
| **OPEN:** | Year-round |
| **SITES:** | 12 |
| **EACH SITE HAS:** | Picnic table, fire ring, lantern post, tent pad |
| **ASSIGNMENT:** | First come, first served; no reservations |
| **REGISTRATION:** | Self-registration on site |
| **FACILITIES:** | Vault toilets, bring your own water |
| **PARKING:** | At campsites only |
| **FEE:** | $7 per night |
| **ELEVATION:** | 900 feet |
| **RESTRICTIONS:** | Pets: On 6-foot leash only Fires: In fire rings only Alcohol: At campsites only Vehicles: Maximum 2 vehicles per site Other: Maximum 14-day stay |

## MAP

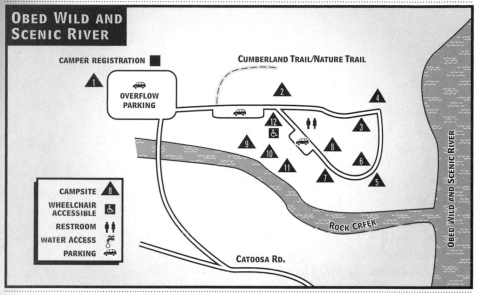

**OBED WILD AND SCENIC RIVER**

CAMPER REGISTRATION

CUMBERLAND TRAIL/NATURE TRAIL

OVERFLOW PARKING

1

2

4

12

3

9

10

8

11

6

7

5

**CAMPSITE** 8
**WHEELCHAIR ACCESSIBLE**
**RESTROOM**
**WATER ACCESS**
**PARKING**

ROCK CREEK

OBED WILD AND SCENIC RIVER

CATOOSA RD.

## GETTING THERE

From the Obed Visitor Center next to the courthouse in downtown Wartburg, take Maiden Street west 2 blocks to Catoosa Road. Turn right onto Catoosa Road and follow it 6 miles to the campground, which is on the right just past the bridge over the Emory River.

starting down Daddy's Creek, where two overlooks await in the first mile. The Rain House, a rock shelter, is a mile farther on. Pick up a trail map and park map at the visitor center in Wartburg. A shorter option is taking the Cumberland Trail up the Emory to a nature trail that leaves right and descends to end at the campground, near the water's edge. No matter which option you choose, grab your tent and head for the Obed.

# OLD FORGE

**O**LD **FORGE WAS THE SITE OF AN** iron forge in the early 1900s. Iron was melted and made into tools for use on the logging railroad that extended up to Cold Springs Mountain. Men cut the timber by hand with crosscut saws then transported the logs via horse or mule before loading them onto trains at the railroad. Talk about hard work! That makes it all the more ironic that this is a recreational site now. It doesn't take much effort nowadays to have a good time at this campground, which was revamped exclusively for tent campers.

The natural setting is appealing. Old Forge is set in a flat along Jennings Creek, which tumbles into numerous falls and pools, some large enough for a swim. Overhead is a mix of hardwoods along with white pine, hemlock, and a little rhododendron. The Forest Service built a wooden fence around the campground with handsome archway entrances. Pass through the archway and follow a gravel path from which little spur trails lead to the walk-in tent campsites. Tent campers are grouped together, while the big-rig campers stay at nearby Horse Creek Campground.

Swing up the flat and pass a few sites that are farther away from the creek but closest to the parking area. Three sites at the head of the flat offer lush solitude. These are ideal campsites for hikers, as they are closest to an archway leading out of the camp onto the Bald Mountain Ridge Scenic Area's trail system. The campground path then swings alongside Jennings Creek, passing the five waterside sites. A couple of spur paths lead down to waterfall overlooks and big pools on the moderate-size stream. One campsite is all by its lonesome self, far down the stream. A vault toilet stands near the camper parking area. You must bring your own water.

> *Old Forge has been melded into a model tenter's campground.*

## RATINGS

Beauty: ✿ ✿ ✿ ✿ ✿
Privacy: ✿ ✿ ✿
Spaciousness: ✿ ✿ ✿ ✿ ✿
Quiet: ✿ ✿ ✿ ✿ ✿
Security: ✿ ✿ ✿
Cleanliness: ✿ ✿ ✿ ✿

**ADDRESS:** 4900 Asheville Highway SR 70 Greeneville, TN 37743

**OPERATED BY:** Forest Service

**INFORMATION:** (423) 638-4108; www.fs.fed.us/r8/cherokee

**OPEN:** Mid-April– mid-December

**SITES:** 10

**EACH SITE HAS:** Picnic table, fire ring, lantern post, tent pad

**ASSIGNMENT:** First come, first served; no reservations

**REGISTRATION:** Self-registration on site

**FACILITIES:** Water spigot, vault toilet

**PARKING:** At tent-camper parking only

**FEE:** $7 per night

**ELEVATION:** 1,920 feet

**RESTRICTIONS:** Pets: On leash only
Fires: In fire rings only
Alcohol: Not allowed
Vehicles: None
Other: Maximum 14-day stay

After setting up camp, check out the campground falls and pools. The waters of Jennings Creek plunge down the rocky face of a rhododendron-choked hollow into surprisingly large pools that invite a dip. Of course there are also trout in there. Licensed anglers can fish both up and downstream for small but scrappy rainbows. Upstream lies the Bald Mountain Ridge Scenic Area. This is my favorite hiking destination in the northern Cherokee National Forest. To explore the streams and hollows of Bald Ridge, pass through the campground archway and cruise up the Jennings Creek Trail to the Little Jennings Creek Trail to reach Round Knob Picnic Area. Turn left onto the Cowbell Hollow Trail and pass through a rich forest to reach the Jennings Creek Trail. Return to camp and complete a 5-mile loop. A more ambitious loop continues on from Round Knob Picnic Area up an old roadbed to reach the Appalachian Trail (A.T.). Turn left on the A.T., straddling the state line to Jerry Cabin Trail shelter. Continue a bit farther to reach Coldsprings Bald, 4,500 feet in elevation. Here you will find a large field affording great views into Tennessee. Watch for the blue blazes to make the left onto the Sarvis Cove Trail. Descend steeply via many switchbacks, then come alongside Sarvis Creek, which has its own pools and cascades. The rhododendron can be thick down here. Reach the more open Poplar Cove Trail and make a left over a dry gap to get to Jennings Creek. Return down Jennings Creek to the camp for a 10-mile day. Less-experienced hikers should consider backtracking from Coldsprings Bald because the Sarvis Cove Trail can be rough and overgrown. Rest assured, a day hike in the Bald Mountains couldn't be near as rough as was a day for those who toiled at Old Forge as loggers. And they didn't return to such a pleasant setting along Jennings Creek as do tent campers today.

# MAP

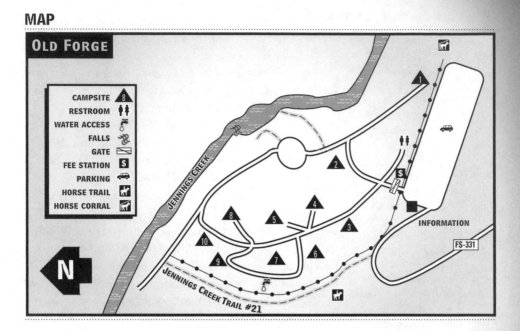

OLD FORGE

| | |
|---|---|
| CAMPSITE | 8 |
| RESTROOM | |
| WATER ACCESS | |
| FALLS | |
| GATE | |
| FEE STATION | S |
| PARKING | |
| HORSE TRAIL | |
| HORSE CORRAL | |

JENNINGS CREEK

JENNINGS CREEK TRAIL #21

INFORMATION

FS-331

N

## GETTING THERE

From Greeneville, take US 11E north to TN 107. Turn right onto TN 107 and follow it east 6.4 miles to Horse Creek Park Road. Turn right onto Horse Creek Park Road and follow it 2.7 miles. (At 0.8 miles Horse Creek Park Road makes a sharp right.) Enter the Cherokee National Forest, then turn right onto Forest Service Road 331 and follow it 2.5 miles to dead-end at Old Forge Campground.

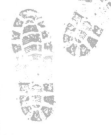

> *Backing up to the Bald Mountains, Paint Creek is well situated for exploring the Greene County Highlands and historic Greeneville, the home of President Andrew Johnson.*

**THE WINDSHIELD WIPERS SQUEAKED** a decidedly unenthusiastic mantra the day we set out for Paint Creek. As we wound down the saturated gravel road, the camping trip seemed more like a job than an outing. But our prospects brightened beyond the small bridge spanning Paint Creek. To our left lay the welcome sight of the Paint Creek Campground. Well laid out on an inside bend of Paint Creek, this cozy campground blends with its surroundings so beautifully that you'll think it was just meant for tent camping. Each campsite is ideally situated among the trees of the forest and is outlined with wood timbers that hold freshly spread gravel, making for an attractive and well-drained site. Eleven of the sites are directly creekside, but there are no bad sites at this campground. They're all large and well separated from one another by thick stands of eastern hemlock, with plenty of room to pitch a tent and spread out a carload of gear.

Two small loops divide the campground. Vault toilets for each sex are unobtrusively placed on each loop. An old-fashioned hand-pump well is located at the campground entrance. There are no electric hookups. The northern loop has only six sites; half are along Paint Creek, a stream worthy of any mountain. The other 15 sites are on the southern loop, which follows Paint Creek as it descends toward the French Broad River.

The early spring sky cleared as we set up camp; the place was our own. After lunch we went for a drive along Forest Service Road 41, which parallels Paint Creek, to see Dudley Falls, which spills into a big pool backed by a rocky bluff. In warm weather, this pool is a popular swimming hole. The road bridges the creek and approaches smaller falls and fishing holes, meandering a few miles to Paint Creek's confluence with the French Broad River at Paint Rock. We scanned the French Broad, cut deep into the mountains. Directly

## RATINGS

Beauty: ✿ ✿ ✿ ✿ ✿
Privacy: ✿ ✿ ✿ ✿
Spaciousness: ✿ ✿ ✿ ✿ ✿
Quiet: ✿ ✿ ✿ ✿
Security: ✿ ✿ ✿
Cleanliness: ✿ ✿ ✿ ✿

across the river lay Huff Island, its banks nearly scoured from high water. The French Broad is a popular canoeing and rafting river. Outfitters are stationed in Del Rio, Tennessee, and across the mountain in Hot Springs, North Carolina.

The Appalachian Trail (A.T.) is easily accessed from Paint Creek. Turn left out of the campground and head 5 miles up FS 31 to Hurricane Gap. The A.T. passes through the gap. Follow the A.T. to your right 0.8 miles up to the Rich Mountain Fire Tower, at an elevation of 3,643 feet. Look down on the French Broad Valley and gaze at the Bald Mountains around you. Mount Mitchell, the highest point east of the Mississippi River at 6,682 feet, is to the east.

On our way home we stopped in Greeneville, established in 1781. A well-preserved town of old brick buildings, its citizens have placed a special emphasis on keeping up the area's many historic sites, including the site of Civil War skirmishes and the home of President Andrew Johnson. Johnson's tenure as president was troubled, starting with his assuming the presidency after Abraham Lincoln's assassination and ending with his nearly being impeached by the Senate during Reconstruction. But the native sons of Greeneville are proud of their president. The National Park Service maintains a visitor center in Greeneville, and the town has undergone a revitalization and restoration of its historic downtown structures. Park your car and check out Johnson's home and tailor shop, the old churches, the Stone Jail, and the Harmony Cemetery.

Remember, if you visit Paint Creek Campground in early spring or late fall, be certain to call ahead to ensure the campground is open.

## KEY INFORMATION

| | |
|---|---|
| **ADDRESS:** | 4900 Asheville Highway SR 70 Greeneville, TN 37743 |
| **OPERATED BY:** | Forest Service |
| **INFORMATION:** | (423) 638-4109; www.fs.fed.us/r8/cherokee |
| **OPEN:** | Mid-April–mid-November |
| **SITES:** | 21 |
| **EACH SITE HAS:** | Fire grate, picnic table, lantern post, tent pad |
| **ASSIGNMENT:** | First come, first served; no reservations |
| **REGISTRATION:** | Self-registration on site |
| **FACILITIES:** | Hand-pumped water, vault toilets |
| **PARKING:** | At campsites only |
| **FEE:** | $10 per night |
| **ELEVATION:** | 1,640 feet |
| **RESTRICTIONS:** | Pets: On 6-foot or shorter leash<br>Fires: In fire grates only<br>Alcohol: At campsites only<br>Vehicles: Trailers up to 26 feet<br>Other: Maximum 14-day stay |

## MAP

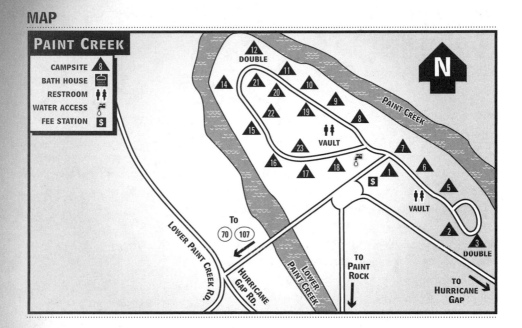

### PAINT CREEK

| | |
|---|---|
| CAMPSITE | 8 |
| BATH HOUSE | |
| RESTROOM | |
| WATER ACCESS | |
| FEE STATION | $ |

12 DOUBLE
11
14
21
20
10
22
9
19
15
8
VAULT
23
7
16
18
17
$
6
1
5
VAULT
2
3 DOUBLE

PAINT CREEK

N

To 70 107

LOWER PAINT CREEK RD.

HURRICANE GAP RD.

LOWER PAINT CREEK

TO PAINT ROCK

TO HURRICANE GAP

## GETTING THERE

From Greeneville, take TN 70 south 12.5 miles. Turn right onto Rollins Chapel Road. Drive 1.1 miles, then turn left onto Lower Paint Creek Road. The pavement ends after 1.1 mile. Continue downhill another 0.5 miles and cross the small bridge over Paint Creek. The Paint Creek Campground is on your left.

# PICKETT STATE PARK

**T**ENNESSEE STATE PARKS come fully loaded with man-made amenities to help you make the most of your visit. But Pickett State Park was already fully loaded with natural features long before it became Tennessee's first state park way back in the 1930s. The campground is vintage, too. It is evident that over the years Pickett's natural beauty, as well as the campground, have passed through caring hands.

> *Tennessee's first state park is 11,750 acres of scenic botanical wonders.*

The main camping area is situated atop a wooded hill. It has the standard circular loop configuration with a road bisecting the center of the loop, making almost a figure eight. You'll climb as you enter the loop. Most sites are on the outer edge of the loop, but the road that bisects the loop also has campsites along it. Tall pines and hardwoods shade the camping area. There is a light understory, mixed with more heavily wooded sections, especially outside the main loop.

The campground was built before RVs existed, so, even though 31 of 32 sites have both water and electricity, it is primarily a tenter's campground. A modern bathhouse with flush toilets and hot showers and a coin laundry are in the very center of the campground. Those staying on the campground's perimeter may have to walk a bit to reach the bathhouse. Speaking of walking, don't forget about the two walk-in tent sites.

Hand-laid stone walls complement the natural surroundings and blend in well with the campground. Even the park water tank is overlaid with stone. The campsites are a bit smaller than normal but offer more than adequate space. It's quiet and secure here in the outer reaches of Fentress County adjacent to the Kentucky state line. A park ranger lives on site at the state park and the park visitor center is nearby.

You may need help figuring out just what to do. Recreational pursuits include tennis, badminton, horseshoes, and volleyball. Any equipment you may need is

## RATINGS

Beauty: ☆ ☆ ☆
Privacy: ☆ ☆ ☆
Spaciousness: ☆ ☆ ☆
Quiet: ☆ ☆ ☆ ☆
Security: ☆ ☆ ☆ ☆ ☆
Cleanliness: ☆ ☆ ☆ ☆

**ADDRESS:** 4605 Pickett Park Highway Jamestown, TN 38556-4141

**OPERATED BY:** Tennessee State Parks

**INFORMATION:** (931) 879-5821; www.tnstateparks.com

**OPEN:** Year-round

**SITES:** 32, plus 2 walk-in tent campsites

**EACH SITE HAS:** Tent pad, fire grate, lantern post, picnic table

**ASSIGNMENT:** First come, first served; no reservations

**REGISTRATION:** At visitor center

**FACILITIES:** Water, flush toilets, showers, laundry, electrical hookups

**PARKING:** At campsites only

**FEE:** $13 per night

**ELEVATION:** 1,500 feet

**RESTRICTIONS:** Pets: On leash only
Fires: In fire grates only
Alcohol: Prohibited
Vehicles: None
Other: Maximum 14-day stay

available free of charge at the park office. Before you imagine this is a wooded health club, let me assure you there's a lot more of the outdoor sort of fun, including a swimming beach open during the summer months at Arch Lake. This 15-acre, S-shaped lake offers trout fishing and canoe and rowboat rentals as well. A park naturalist is on duty during the summer. Headquarters are at the nature center, which is in the middle of the campground. Campfire programs and movies are also part of Pickett's activities.

Finally, there are the landforms, without which no man-made state park could exist. Much of the state forest escaped the logger's ax. Today, more than 58 miles of trails trace beneath the trees, reaching natural bridges, caves, waterfalls, and rock bluffs. The Indian Rockhouse Trail travels 0.2 miles to a huge rock overhang with a water feature in its center. The 2.5-mile Lake Trail Loop crosses Arch Lake on a swinging bridge, then passes a natural bridge before looping back to the picnic area. It is 1 mile down to Double Falls from Thompson Overlook. The Hazard Cave Loop extends 2.5 miles and goes by a sand-floored cave, then by the Natural Bridge, which is more than 80 feet long and 20 feet high.

The two primary park trails are Rock Creek and the Sheltowee Trace–Hidden Passage. The Sheltowee Trace Trail extends 280 miles into Kentucky. Sheltowee means "Big Turtle," which is what the native Indians called Daniel Boone way back when he was adopted into the Shawnee Tribe. The Rock Creek Trail parallels its namesake, passing small waterfalls in a classic, deeply wooded mountain stream. It is 5 miles one way and connects to the Sheltowee Trace Trail. Pickett's master trail is the Hidden Passage Trail, which runs in conjunction with the Sheltowee Trace. The first feature you'll see is a modest arch, then comes the Hidden Passage, a small passageway created by a large rock overhang amid jumbled rocks. Next is Crystal Falls, a delicate three-tiered watery drop. Continuing on down you'll see overlooks and numerous rock houses, some with chestnut benches built by the Civilian Conservation Corps during the Depression. This rewarding loop continues after the Hidden Passage Trail diverges from

# MAP

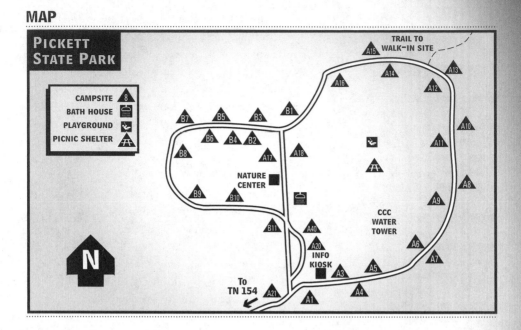

## PICKETT STATE PARK

CAMPSITE
BATH HOUSE
PLAYGROUND
PICNIC SHELTER

TRAIL TO WALK-IN SITE

A15 · A14 · A13 · A12 · A16 · A10 · A11 · A8 · A9

B7 · B5 · B3 · B1 · B6 · B4 · B2 · B8 · A17 · A18

NATURE CENTER

CCC WATER TOWER

B9 · B10 · B11 · A40 · A20 · INFO KIOSK · A6 · A7 · A3 · A5 · A4 · A1

To TN 154

A21

the Sheltowee Trace. Any day hiking here will be a day you'll remember. A rough trail map is available at the visitor center. They'll be glad to help you find a trail to suit you. This is one place where you can stay busy for days with all types of activities. Just make sure to get all your food and supplies back in Jamestown. You'll need the calories.

## GETTING THERE

From Jamestown, take US 127 north 2 miles to TN 154. Turn right on TN 154 and follow it 10 miles. The park entrance will be on your left.

# PRENTICE COOPER STATE FOREST

> *The campground is small but hiking opportunities are big atop the Tennessee River Gorge.*

**P**ERCHED ATOP SUCK CREEK MOUNTAIN, overlooking the Grand Canyon of the Tennessee River, 26,000-acre Prentice Cooper is a surprisingly quiet getaway for nearby Chattanooga residents. It was once the hunting ground of the Cherokees, who lived along the banks of the Tennessee River where Chattanooga now lies. Later, the state took over these once abused lands, which had been selectively logged, then grazed. Now, the state forest is managed for forestry and hunting but also features one of the most spectacular sections of the Cumberland Trail. This forest is also the southern terminus of the trail, which is slated to run the length of the Cumberland Plateau, from the Cumberland Gap National Historic Park, up Kentucky way. Davis Pond campsite is small, with only a couple of developed sites, though at least two other groups could easily squeeze in to the camping area. Set up your camp beside this small, man-made pond and break out the boots to enjoy nearly 40 miles of trails offering far-reaching views from places like Pot Point, set on the rim of the gorge. Mountain bikers can enjoy numerous forest roads that spur off the primary forest road, Tower Road. No matter your mode of exploration, downtown Chattanooga will seem far, far away.

The Davis Pond campsite is the only auto-accessible campsite in the forest. It is situated on a flat of a rib ridge of Suck Creek Mountain. Posts ring the gravel parking area, keeping cars where they belong. On the far side of the posts lies the camping area. It is an alluring grassy spot with scattered shade trees backed by a rising wooded hill. Davis Pond, around one acre in size, forms one border of the campground. To the left, near the campground entrance road, is a vault toilet. Beyond this is the first developed campsite, with a picnic table and rock fire ring. Overhead are shade-casting pines. The other developed site is closer to Davis Pond.

## RATINGS

Beauty: ✿ ✿ ✿ ✿
Privacy: ✿ ✿ ✿
Spaciousness: ✿ ✿ ✿ ✿
Quiet: ✿ ✿ ✿ ✿ ✿
Security: ✿ ✿ ✿ ✿
Cleanliness: ✿ ✿ ✿

Both these sites require a short walk from your car to the camping area. The rest of the campground is suitable for a few other tents, so don't despair if the two sites are taken. There is no water here, only a vault toilet, but there is a pump well at the gated entrance to the state forest. Speaking of this gate, it closes at sunset, and the state forest asks you to be at your campsite by sunset and not to expect to leave until sunrise. This is done to cut down on poaching. Also, be apprised of spring and fall managed hunts in the forest. These hunts are posted on the Web at www.cumberlandtrail.org. Or just call Tennessee Wildlife Resources Agency. Avoid Prentice Cooper on these weekends. During the week, you'll have the state forest to yourself, so get out there and hit the trail. The nearest trailhead is for Pot Point Trail and is back a bit on Tower Road. This trail makes a half-mile run to Snoopers Rock, picking up the Cumberland Trail, then cruises south along the Grand Canyon of the Tennessee River, passing Pot Point and a 30-foot-high natural bridge. More overlooks await before the trail turns up McNabb Gulf and crosses Tower Road, where you can complete your loop. The Mullens Cove Loop is shorter, at 10 miles; it intersects the Cumberland Trail at Indian Rockhouse, then runs the gorge line of the Tennessee River before looping around and up the Mullens Creek Gorge. Other closed jeep roads can make shorter loops for hikers or bikers. No matter what path you take, this mountaintop forest will not fail to please the eye.

## KEY INFORMATION

**ADDRESS:** P.O. Box 160 Hixson, TN 37343

**OPERATED BY:** Tennessee Division of Forestry

**INFORMATION:** (423) 634-3091; www.tn.us/ agriculture/forestry

**OPEN:** Year-round

**SITES:** 4

**EACH SITE HAS:** Picnic table, fire ring

**ASSIGNMENT:** First come, first served; no reservations

**REGISTRATION:** No registration

**FACILITIES:** Vault toilet, bring your own water

**PARKING:** In campground parking area only

**FEE:** None

**ELEVATION:** 1,750 feet

**RESTRICTIONS:** Pets: On 6-foot leash only
Fires: In fire rings only
Alcohol: Prohibited
Vehicles: None
Other: Campers must be at their campsites by sunset; entrance gates are closed from sunset to sunrise.

## MAP

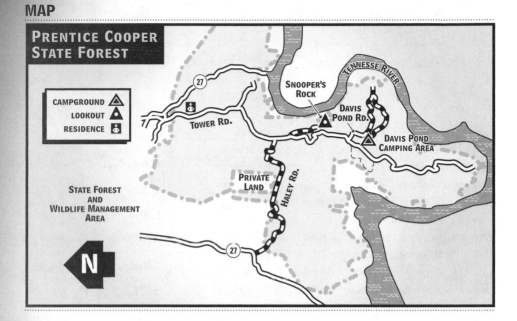

## GETTING THERE

From the junction with Main Street near downtown Chattanooga, take US 27 north 3 miles to US 127 north. Take US 127 north 1.6 miles to TN 27 west. Turn left onto TN 27 west and follow it 8 miles to Choctow Trace Road. Turn left here and go 0.2 miles to reach Game Reserve Road. Turn left and enter Prentice Cooper State Forest, where it becomes Tower Road. Continue on Tower Road 7 miles to reach Davis Pond Road. Turn left onto Davis Pond Road and follow it 0.6 miles to reach the campground, on your left.

# ROCK CREEK

*Erwin*

**B**ACK IN THE **1930S,** the Civilian Conservation Corps (CCC) developed the Rock Creek area for forest recreation, and Rock Creek Campground is one result of these Depression-era work projects. As an antidote for an ailing economy, the Corps was assembled to provide jobs for unemployed men. Detractors of the organization accused the CCC of doing "make-work." Here at Rock Creek, the Corps introduced the works of man into the wilds of East Tennessee to make the Cherokee National Forest more enjoyable for visitors. What a fine area they had to start with! The national forest is laden with virgin timberland and clear mountain streams that nestle against the backbone of the Unaka Mountains. Of course, the Forest Service has improved and maintained the area since the days of the Corps. But the old-time feel remains, as well as most of the original infrastructure. Today, as then, we can camp in the cool, shady cove of Rock Creek.

The campground is arranged in three loops. Mother Nature landscaped this place well, with tall hardwoods looming over a thick understory of moss, ferns, rhododendron, and small trees amid gray boulders. Rock Creek Campground has a deep-woods feel. The farther back you go in the cove, the more this is evident. The white noise of Rock Creek is your constant companion here. Loop A has ten sites, each with a parking area large enough to accommodate an RV. Two Loop A sites are for group camping. Loop B has 11 sites, including 3 double sites. Loops A and B both offer electrical hookups and share a modern bathhouse with flush toilets and warm showers. Loop C is located farthest back in the cove, against a steep hill. It has a very thick understory for maximum privacy. Its 13 sites are ideally suited for tent campers. Farther up from Loop C are four walk-in tent sites. There are two campground hosts.

> *Camp in the cool and Shady Rock Creek Campground adjacent to the impressive Unaka Mountain Wilderness.*

## RATINGS

Beauty: ✪ ✪ ✪ ✪ ✪
Privacy: ✪ ✪ ✪ ✪
Spaciousness: ✪ ✪ ✪ ✪
Quiet: ✪ ✪ ✪ ✪ ✪
Security: ✪ ✪ ✪ ✪
Cleanliness: ✪ ✪ ✪ ✪

## KEY INFORMATION

**ADDRESS:** 4900 Asheville Highway SR 70 Greeneville, TN 37743

**OPERATED BY:** Forest Service

**INFORMATION:** (423) 638-4109; www.fs.fed.us/r8/ cherokee

**OPEN:** May–October

**SITES:** 32, plus 4 walk-in tent sites

**EACH SITE HAS:** Tent pad, lantern post, picnic table, fire pit

**ASSIGNMENT:** First come, first served; no reservations

**REGISTRATION:** Self-registration on site

**FACILITIES:** Water, warm showers, flush toilets, swimming pool

**PARKING:** At individual sites

**FEE:** $15–$30 per night, $10 per night walk-in tent sites

**ELEVATION:** 2,350 feet

**RESTRICTIONS:** Pets: On leash only
Fires: In fire rings only
Alcohol: Prohibited
Vehicles: None
Other: Maximum 14-day stay

One of the most intriguing features of Rock Creek Recreation Area is the swimming pool. Another product of the CCC's efforts, the pool is a concrete-and-rock-lined basin of clear stream water, lying behind a small dam. A creek runs into the head of the pool, which is circled by a walkway. Trout will be swimming with you. The Rock Creek Trail parallels its namesake, passing small waterfalls in a classic, deeply wooded mountain stream. A bathhouse with changing rooms, rest rooms, and showers for each sex is nearby. The day was a bit cool for a swim during our visit, but some hardy youngsters were splashing about and having a good time.

Maybe you should save your swim until after a scenic hike in the Unaka Mountain Wilderness that borders the campground. Leave your vehicle at the campsite and depart directly from the campground. The Rattlesnake Ridge Trail (Forest Trail 26) climbs east 3 miles to the Pleasant Garden Overlook at 4,800 feet. At the base of Unaka Mountain is Rock Creek Falls. FT 26 leads out of the campground along the creek. A few creek crossings later, the falls' multiple descents come into view beneath the forest canopy—there is always something relaxing about a cascade. This hike is 2.3 miles one way. Other short hikes leave from the campground. Take the 0.4-mile Hemlock Forest Trail Loop and find out about this important component of the Southern Appalachian woodlands. Then, walk the 0.2-mile Trail of the Hardwoods Loop for comparison's sake.

Bicyclists have the 0.8-mile Rock Creek Bicycle Trail to enjoy as well. For any supplies you may need, Erwin is less than 4 miles away. However, it feels like civilization is light years away at Rock Creek Campground and the Unaka Wilderness.

## MAP

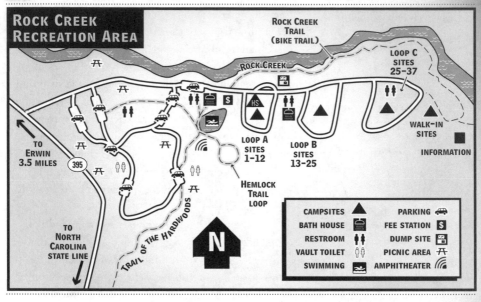

**ROCK CREEK RECREATION AREA**

ROCK CREEK TRAIL (BIKE TRAIL)

ROCK CREEK

LOOP C SITES 25-37

TO ERWIN 3.5 MILES

395

TO NORTH CAROLINA STATE LINE

TRAIL OF THE HARDWOODS

N

LOOP A SITES 1-12

HEMLOCK TRAIL LOOP

LOOP B SITES 13-25

HS

WALK-IN SITES

INFORMATION

| | | | |
|---|---|---|---|
| CAMPSITES | ▲ | PARKING | 🚐 |
| BATH HOUSE | | FEE STATION | $ |
| RESTROOM | 👫 | DUMP SITE | |
| VAULT TOILET | 👤👤 | PICNIC AREA | 🪑 |
| SWIMMING | | AMPHITHEATER | |

## GETTING THERE

From Erwin take TN 395 east 3.1 miles. Turn left into the Rock Creek Recreation Area. The campground will be on your right.

# ROUND MOUNTAIN

> *Enjoy the mountain meadow of Max Patch and lofty wooded camping.*

**ROUND MOUNTAIN CAMPGROUND** is off the beaten path in a seemingly forgotten corner of the Bald Mountains in Cherokee National Forest. Maybe it is the tortuously twisting gravel road that keeps most visitors away. We stayed here on a Friday night with good weather in mid-June, and only 3 of the 14 sites were occupied. The three other groups were tent campers. Those who find Round Mountain will relish the tranquil high-country campground that is so in tune with the woods that it seems to have been constructed by Mother Nature.

Round Mountain's sites are spaced along a single, thickly forested loop road that is bordered in moss— you are literally in the woods. Tall trees, including high-elevation species such as yellow birch and pin cherry, intermingle with hemlock and white pine to provide a thick overhead canopy, shading all campers and the loop road. A junglelike growth of rhododendron on the forest floor separates the campsites. Noisy little streams cascade down the mountainside amid the brush.

The first two sites are actually picnic sites and are located on the approach road to the loop. The next five sites are placed among large trees and dense undergrowth. You must climb some steps to reach the campground's most isolated site. One other walk-up site is available. There are additional sites along the loop, where they blend in well with the scenery and feature plenty of distance between each other for maximum privacy. A traditional hand-pump well provides cool mountain water. The pump is located at the beginning of the loop, along with a comfort station with clean vault toilets for each sex. Make your last supply stop in Newport and don't plan on coming off Round Mountain until your stay is over. That winding road to and from civilization is a bear. Also, be certain

## RATINGS

Beauty: ✩ ✩ ✩ ✩ ✩
Privacy: ✩ ✩ ✩ ✩ ✩
Spaciousness: ✩ ✩ ✩ ✩
Quiet: ✩ ✩ ✩ ✩ ✩
Security: ✩ ✩ ✩
Cleanliness: ✩ ✩ ✩ ✩

to call ahead to verify that the campground is open if you plan to visit in early spring or late fall.

It is just a short distance from the campground to the Walnut Mountain Trail. Walk out to Forest Service Road 107, then go downhill 30 yards to reach the trailhead. It leads 1 mile to Rattlesnake Gap and another mile to the Appalachian Trail near the Walnut Mountain shelter. There will be attractive scenery regardless of which way you turn on the A.T.

Our June journey took place on a cool mountain morning. Sunlight penetrated the forest canopy here and there, illuminating a light mist that rose from the woodland floor. The famed Max Patch was waiting. We turned left out of the campground onto FS 107, motoring 2 miles up to Lemon Gap and the North Carolina border. The Appalachian Trail threaded through these lovely groves, as it does in so many of the Southern Appalachians' treasure spots. On we drove, veering right at Lemon Gap onto FS 1182 and driving 3.5 miles farther, past a trout pond maintained by the Pisgah National Forest. Old-timers in overalls lounged in lawn chairs beside the pond, fishing poles in hand.

Beyond the pond, the forest opened to our left, revealing Max Patch in all its glory. The 230-acre field was once part of a working farm; the field now supports only wildflowers, which bloomed by the thousands, all facing the morning sun. We crested the top of the field at 4,629 feet and were rewarded with a 360-degree view. To the south stood the Great Smoky Mountains. Mount Sterling, with its metal fire tower, and Mount Cammerer, with its distinctive stone tower, stood out among the countless peaks. The open fields of the Bald Mountains stretched out to the north. It seemed as if we were in the very heart of the Southern Appalachians. We may have been.

Round Mountain is my favorite campground in this entire guidebook. Between the quiet solitude and classic, high-country atmosphere of each campsite, and the magnificence of Max Patch, this area exudes the best of the uplands that extend from the North Woods into Dixie. It is hard to go wrong combining the beauty of the Appalachians and the charm of the South.

## KEY INFORMATION

**ADDRESS:** 4900 Asheville Highway SR 70 Greeneville, TN 37743

**OPERATED BY:** Forest Service

**INFORMATION:** (423) 638-4109; www.fs.fcd.us/r8/cherokee

**OPEN:** Mid-April–mid-December

**SITES:** 14

**EACH SITE HAS:** Tent pad, fire grate, lantern post, picnic table, stand-up grill

**ASSIGNMENT:** First come, first served; no reservations

**REGISTRATION:** Self-registration on site

**FACILITIES:** Hand-pumped water, vault toilets

**PARKING:** At campsites only

**FEE:** $7 per night

**ELEVATION:** 3,000 feet

**RESTRICTIONS:** Pets: On 6-foot or shorter leash
Fires: In fire grates only
Alcohol: At campsites only
Vehicles: 22-foot trailer limit
Other: Maximum 14-day stay

# MAP

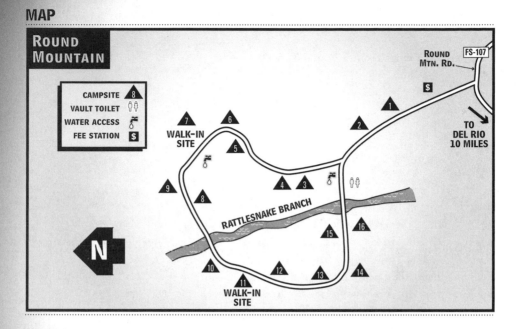

## ROUND MOUNTAIN

| | |
|---|---|
| CAMPSITE | 8 |
| VAULT TOILET | 👥 |
| WATER ACCESS | 🚰 |
| FEE STATION | $ |

ROUND MTN. RD. — FS-107

TO DEL RIO 10 MILES

WALK-IN SITE

RATTLESNAKE BRANCH

WALK-IN SITE

N

## GETTING THERE

From Newport, take US 25/70 about 10 miles to TN 107 at Del Rio. Turn right on TN 107 and follow it 5.8 miles. Turn left on gravel FS 107 (Round Mountain Road) as it climbs Round Mountain. After 6 miles, Round Mountain Campground will be on your left.

# SYLCO

**I**F YOU PLACE A HIGH PRIORITY on quiet solitude and close-at-hand wilderness hiking, Sylco is just the place for you. It is located in an isolated area of the Cherokee National Forest in the extreme south-eastern corner of Tennessee. You don't have to worry about RVs or trailers coming to this campground. There are three ways to get in here and they're all rough and remote, just like the Sylco area. You'll follow these roads, then out of nowhere, in the middle of nowhere, will appear a grassy plot of land interspersed with shade trees and picnic tables! Just make sure you have your supplies with you.

Primarily used as a hunting camp in fall, this campground is very lightly used the rest of the year. It is so lightly used in fact that the Forest Service doesn't even charge campers to stay here! And only a few of the 12 sites appear to get enough use to even beat down the grass that grows around the picnic tables.

It's remote—no registration and no campground hosts. Some sites don't even have both a picnic table and grill; some just have a fire ring with the table. There's even one grill with no table. You'll find no tent pads either. Just pitch your tent right on the grass; it may slope a bit. This is the most primitive campground in this guidebook. Not to say this place is ragged and neglected, it's just remote—and clean. Surrounded by second-growth forest, the campground is in a dry, mid-mountain slope area that has been selectively cleared of trees, leaving tall oaks and pines to partially shade the grassy campsites below. There's no understory between the spacious and open sites to shield you from other campers, but there probably won't be any other campers—you'll have wild animals for company, and birds will be your noisy neighbors.

This lightly used campground extends onto both sides of the road. A short loop swings by the four sites

> *Sylco, near Big Frog and Cohutta wildernesses, is the most primitive campground profiled in this book.*

## RATINGS

Beauty: ✪ ✪ ✪
Privacy: ✪ ✪ ✪
Spaciousness: ✪ ✪ ✪ ✪ ✪
Quiet: ✪ ✪ ✪ ✪
Security: ✪ ✪
Cleanliness: ✪ ✪ ✪

## KEY INFORMATION

| | |
|---|---|
| **ADDRESS:** | 3171 US 64 Benton, TN 37370 |
| **OPERATED BY:** | Forest Service |
| **INFORMATION:** | (423) 338-5201; www.fs.fed.us/r8/cherokee |
| **OPEN:** | Year-round |
| **SITES:** | 12, with 9 more on the Conasauga River |
| **EACH SITE HAS:** | Picnic table, grill |
| **ASSIGNMENT:** | First come, first served; no reservations |
| **REGISTRATION:** | Not necessary |
| **FACILITIES:** | Vault toilet |
| **PARKING:** | At campsites |
| **FEE:** | None |
| **ELEVATION:** | 1,200 feet |
| **RESTRICTIONS:** | Pets: On leash only Fires: In fire rings only Alcohol: Not allowed Vehicles: Parking at sites only |

on the downslope. Their tables are fairly close together, so the sites could be suitable for a group camp. A larger loop circles around the upper eight sites. All but one of the sites are in the center of the loop. None of the sites have an official parking spur. Pull over to one side of the loop or just park in the grass. Only two of the sites appear to have been used in recent years, and they have parking areas. A vault toilet for each sex stands at the high point of the upper loop.

The campground has no Forest Service–provided water. But nature will provide you with some in case you left yours behind. A narrow path leads 75 yards downslope from the lowest picnic table of the lower loop to a small clear stream. To be on the safe side, treat or boil this water. The Forest Service has developed some primitive campsites on the banks of the Conasauga River, 3 miles south down Forest Service Road 221. These nine sites are free and are actually in better shape than those at Sylco. A vault toilet is the only amenity down here.

Sylco makes a great base camp for the area's wilderness hiking, trout and smallmouth bass fishing, and forest drives. But you'll need a Forest Service map of the Cherokee to make your way around. Big Frog and Cohutta form a 45,000-acre wilderness area (plenty of room for a bear or two). Three miles south of Sylco is Jacks River and the Cohutta Wilderness in Georgia. The Jacks River Trail (Forest Trail 13) follows an old railroad bed, crossing Jacks River many times. Look for rotting crossties and old railroad spikes. Trout and some especially aggressive smallmouth bass dwell here. The 8-mile hike to Jacks River Falls is worth the 20 fords.

If you like the view from up high, take one of the trails that lead to the top of Big Frog Mountain (4,224 feet), the centerpiece of the Big Frog Wilderness. The Chestnut Mountain Trail (Forest Trail 63) climbs the mountain connecting the Wolf Ridge Trail for a 3.7-mile hike to the mountaintop. Another fine route uses Big Creek Trail (Forest Trail 68) connecting to Barkleggin Trail then to Big Frog via Big Frog Trail. Big Creek offers high-quality trout fishing as well. Excellent forest drives loop back to Sylco. No four-wheel-drive vehicles are necessary. Peavine Road (Forest Service Road 221)

## MAP

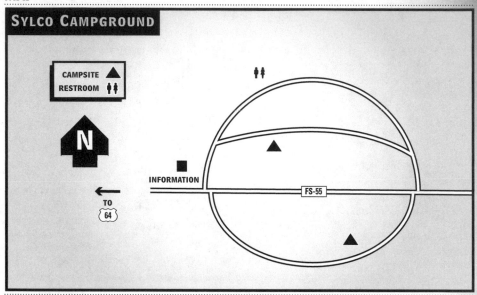

**SYLCO CAMPGROUND**

CAMPSITE ▲
RESTROOM ♂♀

N

■ INFORMATION

FS-55

← TO (64)

leads back to US 64 and the famed Ocoee River. Big Frog Road (FS 62) skirts Big Frog and Cohutta wildernesses, offering you a taste of the wild without making you leave your vehicle. Go slow, ignore the bumps, and try to keep your eyes on the road as well as the scenery. Afterward you can return to your primitive campground at Sylco.

## GETTING THERE

From Benton, drive 2 miles south on US 411 to US 64. Take US 64 east 6 miles to the Ocoee District Ranger Station. Buy a map of the Cherokee National Forest! From the ranger station, take US 64 west 4.9 miles. Turn left onto Cookson Creek/Baker's Creek Road and go 3.5 miles to the national forest boundary; at the boundary, Baker's Creek Road becomes FS 55. Continue 6.5 miles on FS 55 to Sylco.

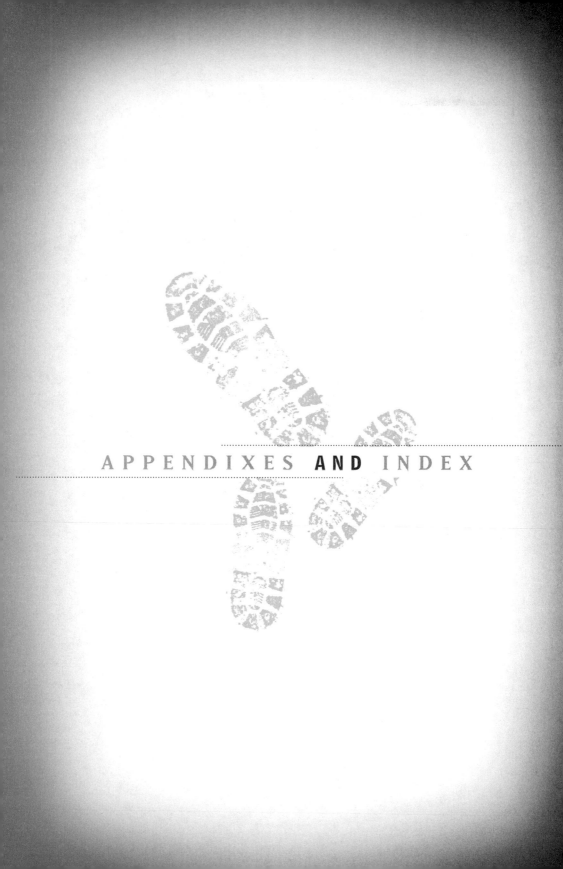

APPENDIXES **AND** INDEX

# APPENDIX A
# CAMPING EQUIPMENT CHECKLIST

The basic utensils and smaller items I routinely use on camping trips are conveniently packed in a large storage bin that transfers easily from garage to car in seconds. It makes preparing for a camping trip efficient. All I have to do is grab a tent and sleeping bag, gather food to bring, and away I go. If I don't have it when I get to my campsite, I figure I really didn't need it in the first place. Some of the basic items I do carry are:

## COOKING UTENSILS
Bottle opener/corkscrew
Coffee pot
Containers of salt, pepper, other favorite
    seasonings, cooking oil, sugar
Cups, dishes, bowls
Dish soap (biodegradable)
Frying pan (cast iron)
Fuel for campstove
Large water container
Lighter, matches, etc.
Pots with lids (at least two, large and
    medium)
Small campstove
Tin foil
Utensils, including big spoon, spatula,
    paring knife

## FIRST-AID KIT
Antibiotic cream
Aspirin
Band-Aids, assorted sizes
Benadryl
Gauze pads
Insect repellent
Moleskin
Personal medications, clearly marked
Sunscreen/lip balm

## SLEEPING GEAR
Pillow
Sleeping bag and liner (optional)
Sleeping pad (inflatable or insulated)
Tent with tub floor; tent fly, ground tarp

## MISCELLANEOUS
Bath soap (biodegradable)
Camera and film
Camp chair
Candles
Cooler
Deck of cards
Duct tape
Fire starter
Flashlight or headlamp with fresh batteries
Foul-weather clothing
Paper towels
Plastic zip-top bags
Sunglasses
Toilet paper
Water bottle
Wool blanket

## OPTIONAL
Barbecue grill
Binoculars (waterproof)
Field guides
Fishing gear
GPS unit
Lantern or tent candles
Maps, charts, other references

# APPENDIX B
# SOURCES OF
# INFORMATION

**CHEROKEE NATIONAL FOREST**
2800 North Ocoee Street
P.O. Box 2010
Cleveland, TN 37320
www.fs.fed.us/r8/cherokee

**BIG SOUTH FORK NATIONAL RIVER
AND RECREATION AREA**
4564 Leatherwood Road
Oneida, TN 37841
(931) 879-4890
www.nps.gov/biso

**GREAT SMOKY MOUNTAINS
NATIONAL PARK**
107 Park Headquarters Road
Gatlinburg, TN 37320
(865) 436-1200
www.nps.gov/grsm

**LAND BETWEEN THE LAKES NATIONAL
RECREATION AREA**
100 Van Morgan Drive
Golden Pond, KY 42211
(800) LBL-7077
www.lbl.org

**NATCHEZ TRACE PARKWAY**
2680 Natchez Trace Parkway
Tupelo, MS 38801
(800) 305-7417
www.nps.gov/natr

**TENNESSEE DEPARTMENT OF TOURISM**
Rachel Jackson State Office Building
320 Sixth Avenue, Fifth Floor
Nashville, TN 37243
(800) GO2-TENN
www.tnvacation.com

**TENNESSEE STATE PARKS**
Seventh Floor, L&C Tower
401 Church Street
Nashville, TN 37243
(888) 867-2757
www.tnstateparks.com

**U.S. ARMY CORPS OF ENGINEERS**
U.S. Army Corps of Engineers
Nashville District
P.O. Box 1070
Nashville, TN 37202
(615) 736-7161
www.lrn.usace.army.mil

# INDEX

# ABOUT THE AUTHOR

**J**OHNNY **M**OLLOY **IS AN OUTDOOR WRITER** based in Johnson City, Tennessee. A native Tennessean, he was born in Memphis and moved to Knoxville in 1980 to attend the University of Tennessee. It was in the Great Smoky Mountains National Park that he developed his love of the natural world, which has become the primary focus of his life. Molloy has averaged over 100 nights in the wild per year since the early 1980s, backpacking, canoeing, and camping throughout our country. He has spent over 650 nights in the Smokies alone, where he cultivated his woodsmanship and expertise on those lofty mountains.

Now Molloy employs his love of the outdoors in his occupation. The results of his efforts are both guidebooks and true-adventure storybooks whose action takes place throughout the United States from Florida to Wisconsin to Colorado and many points in between. Molloy has also written numerous articles for magazines and Web sites. He continues to write to this day and to travel extensively to all four corners of the United States, pursuing a variety of outdoor activities. For Johnny Molloy's latest news, please visit **www.johnnymolloy.com.**